Francis Ruiter

OUT
OF MY
MIND

In Love with Life

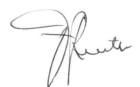

Out Of My Mind: In Love with Life
Copyright © 2012 by Francis Ruiter

ISBN: 978-1-77069-435-4

Word Alive Press
131 Cordite Road, Winnipeg, MB R3W 1S1
www.wordalivepress.ca

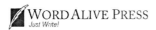

Library and Archives Canada Cataloguing in Publication

Ruiter, Francis, 1929-
    Out of my mind : in love with life / Francis Ruiter.

ISBN 978-1-77069-435-4

    1. Ruiter, Francis, 1929-. 2. Dutch Canadians--Biography.
3. Alzheimer's disease--Patients--Canada--Biography.
4. Immigrants--Canada--Biography. I. Title.

FC106.D9Z7 2012   971'.00439310092   C2012-900662-9

I dedicate this book to my wife Grace
and three daughters,
Linda, Carolyn and Marianne,
and my grandchildren.

Contents

Part Two: Poems

Part One: Short Stories

Joy Ride 1945

By the time the war ended I was 16 years old. Not only did I celebrate the end of the war, I rejoiced that I was finally old enough to get my driver's license. Getting my license was one of the highlights of the year and I could barely wait to jump on a motorbike. I remember one evening I wanted to show off my skills so I asked a hired field worker if he would care to join me on a bike ride. He agreed and his excitement was fuelled by the notion that this would be his first ride ever on a motorbike.

My passenger was somewhat apprehensive climbing onto the back seat, but did not want to miss out on the excitement. I took the main road along the dike that overlooks the Zuider Zee heading for the nearby town of Enkhuizen, a 17th century seaport.

Electricity was still scarce so the darkness covered us like a blanket as we entered Enkhuizen. Suddenly a bright, red light appeared out of nowhere and I realized the local constable was doing his duty. Since I did not have the required documents with me I decided to evade him by first slowing down, then gunning the engine and making an abrupt turn into a side street, crossing over a small bridge spanning a canal and turning my headlights off.

I could see the policeman trying to pursue me on his bicycle. My motorized vehicle surpassed his mode of transportation by miles. Meanwhile, my passenger, although a little scared, hooted with the thrill of adventure. I had to make a decision but the options were few. It wouldn't be easy hiding from the law because there were very few motorized vehicles around after the war. Someone was bound to notice two rascals on a motorbike. All the constable need do was to "ask around!" We needed a stratgey.

Rather than making a long detour and risk meeting up with other policemen I decided to circle around the city at low speed so as not to make much noise. Hopefully the officer would still be searching in the other direction. Sure enough, I got away without being discovered so I high-tailed it for home. My friend on the rear saddle had the thrill of his life and lots to talk about with his fellow workers.

A week later I went for another ride through our own village but still had not located the necessary documents – I had actually forgotten to search for them. On my way home from this trip I spied that same constable standing with his bicycle under a street light in my neighbourhood. He waved his flashlight for me to stop. I thought: once lucky, twice smart. I acted on impulsc foolishly. I should have known that the local cop knew everybody in town and also knew who owned a motorcycle. As I took off he followed me to my home. Realizing that was not the place to be, I headed for my brother's house to see if he might know where those missing papers were to operate a motor vehicle. Meanwhile, the policemen went to our home and gave my mother an earful.

My brother lived half a mile down the road from us. I asked him about those lost papers. He did not know where they were so after stalling for as long as I could, I headed out.

I had barely left my brother's place in the general direction of home, when red lights began flashing. I knew I was in deep trouble. No use trying to evade him this time around. I was nabbed. The constable had another officer with him who was watching from the opposite direction just in case I tried to get away again.

My uniformed friend was not very happy with me, to say the least. His bulging, crimson face spewed forth vulgarities and a reprimand that remains forever etched in my brain. He tossed the book at me: charging me with five offences. Eventually he allowed me to go home, but I was required to appear at the police station the following morning to produce the necessary documents.

Before making a full confession to my father, I talked to my younger brother who told me that the police officer had stormed into our home the night before demanding to know my whereabouts.

My father, bless his heart, kept his cool and counseled me on how to proceed with the charges against me. He helped me locate the paperwork I needed, then told me to be remorseful and to apologize profusely to the officer for my careless behavior.

I took my father's sage advice, hoping to minimize the serious charges. The officer had cooled down considerably. After letting me have my say and hearing my apology, he withdrew two of the five charges which meant I would not have to go to court. I figured he was probably sparing my father the embarrassment. I was one relieved young man...

Lesson for the day: Don't try to be a smart-aleck and don't push my luck!

Summer Wine in 1951

In my Ford pickup truck on a Friday afternoon Peter, my cousin, and I headed home, heaving left of the sawmill where we were employed. Before leaving, a fellow worker, Harry, asked me if I could get him a half-gallon of wine while I was in town and bring it to him when returning on Sunday night. "Sure; sure. No problem," I said.

Peter and I stayed overnight with his parents. I bought the wine on Saturday morning and hid it in a space behind the seat of my Ford. On Sunday morning after attending a church service, we enjoyed a delicious meal of potato and fresh vegetables. At Peter's parents place. After the meal Peter's parents took a nap. Then being a sunny afternoon, Pete and his brother John decided to go for a drive in my pickup truck.

We headed for an open bush area a few miles away from the farm to enjoy the scenery. It was hot inside the truck and we were getting thirsty. We wondered where we might get a drink of water to quench our thirst. Then I remembered that I had a half-gallon of wine behind the seat of the truck and asked if they would like a sip. I explained Harry's request, then I shrugged and decided we could have a little taste. I figured our friend Harry wouldn't mind. We reasoned that we could share the cost of the wine with him when we get back to the sawmill on Sunday night.

Under the shade of a few trees, sitting in my truck, we took a taste and tasted some more. Birds flew around the area, chasing flies; you could not find a better day to enjoy the scenery and discuss nonsense.

Then, suddenly, two other fellows we were acquainted with showed up. I hid the wine when I saw them coming toward us, but when they got close we started a conversation. One of them took a whiff of us and asked what we were drinking. We smiled sheepishly and had to admit that we'd had a few drinks. "Well, what about your friends? Don't we get a taste?" "Well, okay," I said, "take one draw but we have to save some for Harry." So they took a draw: they found it tasty and took another draw.

Our bottle was not labeled. We tried to identify what kind of wine it was but gave up. It just tasted good. Then, when I checked the contents of the bottle, it seemed close to being empty. I suggested finishing it, saying I would tell Harry that I accidentally dropped it and we would get him another one.

By then it was teatime at my uncle's place and they expected us to attend the Sunday afternoon church service. We worried about the wine on our breath. We discussed whether we should go to church or not, but we knew if we didn't we'd be questioned. It would be better to go and just try to keep our faces turned away from our elders.

I took my Uncle and Aunt in my truck to the church, while my cousins took their two sisters with them in their car. Fortunately it was still warm outside so I kept my window open and my face away from them.

Arriving at the church, John and I sat down a few benches ahead of his parents.

We felt comfortable at first, but the wine was still working in our system and the alcohol was causing an equilibrium problem. We were swaying in our bench.

When it came to singing, we discovered our balance was a bit off. By the end of the service, the room had heated up. We had to sing one more song. John got up, but was swaying. I stood close to him, to keep him upright. Fortunately, he was singing with a loud voice, "When the roll is called up yonder..." which showed his devotedness and saved us from the congregation discovering we were tipsy.

When we arrived back at the sawmill Harry was waiting for us, ready to taste the wine that same night. We apologized sincerely, and promised to get him some more later. He called us skunks and we really were!

Smoking Cigarettes

"My first taste of a cigarette was at a tender age of fourteen even with the war in 1943 in Holland making them a real scarcity at the time. All it really took was a few leaves rolled up in some snatched cigarette papers and I was off!"

Sticking the crudely rolled cigarette between my lips as I had seen my older brothers do, I inhaled several deep draws of the nicotine. I did not like the taste and the cigarette made me dizzy. I had been charged with pulling weeds in the garden in front of our home, but I was so dizzy that I lay down between some shrubs, slept for an hour, and awoke feeling sick.

That incident cured me of cigarettes for a couple of years but, when I reached 16years of age, I considered myself a man and, in my day, men smoked. After I accumulated a few dimes I bought my first package of tobacco, which I rolled into cigarette paper. I didn't smoke very often at first. I worked in the fields with other employees who were older and when we stopped working for a rest period, they lighted up and I would join them. Gradually, however, I got used to the tobacco and I made myself believe that it tasted good.

When it was one of my parent's birthdays, my uncles and aunts would gather in our spacious living room. Cigarettes and cigars would be on the table for anyone of age to help themselves and, before an hour went by, the room was full of smoke. A door or window would likely be kept open, but the smoke was still thick. It was part of our culture and we did not know that smoking could hinder our health.

On Sundays, after the church service ended, some men would light up a cigarette as soon as they reached the exit door from the upper balcony: a practice not much appreciated by most parishes.

Fortunately, women did not smoke in those days, but this did not save them from the damaging effects of inhaled second hand smoke from the men who smoked in their homes. Everyone accepted this practice as normal.

As time went by, I became more and more addicted to the nicotine.

My wife, who kept our house spotless, was washing the windows one day and I asked her why. "The windows get dirty from you and others smoking in our home," she said. Sure enough, when I looked carefully, I could see yellow-tinted windows and curtains.

One time, while traveling several hours on dusty gravel roads and lighting up a cigarette every ten minutes, my mouth became dry and it got really stinky in the car. I had to tell myself to wait until I had covered another 50 kilometer before lighting up another cigarette. At this time I was thinking about quitting smoking.

Nicotine had become an addictive substance and it had also become an unconscious habit. I used to grab a cigarette without really thinking, as my fingers seemed to look for something to hold on to.

I remember, too, coming home one night after having an altercation in a church meeting with my Pastor, and I was very upset. I was still upset when I went to bed and I could not sleep. I had to get up and have a cigarette, but found that I did not have any left. I promptly got into my car at midnight to find a place where I could buy some. My wife wondered if I had gone back to my Pastor to have it out with him.

My young school-aged children came home one day and told me that their teacher said that smoking is bad for a person and that smoke in the house was bad for the children too. My, oh my! I knew the teacher was right. I admitted to my children that it was a bad habit and that I should quit smoking soon.

Actually, I had come to the same conclusion a few years earlier and managed to quit for a couple of months; that is, until I made a trip to Holland for my parent's anniversary. Everybody smoked at the party and I reasoned that I could handle the odd cigarette without too much difficulty. However, I'd fooled myself. I ended up buying a packet of cigarettes initially just to be able to share them with family members and other guests who had also shared their cigarettes with me. Later, flying home with a packet of Marlboro cigarettes in my jacket, I lit one up a few times. After all, it was such a long trip I figured, and when I got home I could handle my smoking habit and quit for sure.

Needless to say, it became a bad habit again. So, when my two older daughters asked me why I smoked, that smoking was bad for our health, I promised I would quit soon. Even with good intentions, though, I kept smoking for some time.

As an insurance agent, I made frequent calls to prospective clients after supper. Often I'd make calls without setting up an appointment for fear that people would brush me off. It was better to talk to people in person. Before knocking on their doors, I would extinguish my cigarette.

If they were not at home, I went back to my car and reached for my cigarettes again. My mouth was often dry and my breath smelled dirty. I would talk to myself. "What is it with you Francis? What are your plans? Stick with the stinking cigarettes or come clean and be a man who can live up to promises you made to your wife and children?" I prayed about my struggle, desperately wanting to stop my smoking habit. It was now or never.

Around that time, I became a member of the YMCA where I would swim four times a week. I also took up running, encouraged by a friend. It was going pretty good and I considered running in marathons. I realized that if I planned to go into competition, my body would need a lot of oxygen. That was the clincher.

From there on in, each hour, when my mind said it was time for a smoke, I would counter with a firm, "No, I quit! Go behind me, devil." Each time my body or mind was telling me I needed a smoke, I'd fight back. "Don't lie to me," I would say to myself. "I don't want it!" To make it even harder to succumb to temptation, I made sure I did not have any cigarettes on hand anymore. Though it was difficult not to accept a cigarette from a friendly person, gradually, over time, I won the fight. Hourly battles became half days and then full days of relative freedom from craving, until several months passed and the nicotine in my system was gone and I finally felt safe.

I was never to smoke again. However, interestingly, one night I was dreaming about riding a horse I had ridden many years ago. In the dream I sat in the saddle with a cigarette hanging out of my mouth. Suddenly I realized I was not a smoker anymore when I said to myself, "Oh well, just once in memory of riding that old horse!"

Another incident several months later is also a vivid memory. I'd gone for lunch with some friends when someone offered me a cigarette. Without thinking, I accepted it. Then when he offered to light it, I almost screamed and said, "No! I do not smoke!" They looked at me and apologized, saying they'd forgotten. That was a close call.

I was 16 when I started smoking and 37 when I finally quit!

The Cowboy

One of my boyhood dreams was to become a cowboy and roam wide-open spaces on my trusty steed. So, in 1948 when I immigrated to Canada from Holland, it seemed my vision might just become a reality.

As I sought out a job as a ranch hand in this expansive and wonderful new country, I was determined to learn the ropes and become a full-fledged "Canadian Cowboy." I was more than excited to discover my very own uncle needed some help on his ranch in Houston, British Columbia. He hired me on and soon I became familiar with horses and cattle drives, cowboy lingo and how to dress the part. Before long I fancied myself a real cowboy.

In 1967, my parents sent an invitation to attend their 55th wedding anniversary back in Holland. The opportunity to show myself off to my family in my new position had finally presented itself. I had it in mind to demonstrate to my not-so-well-informed European clan what a cowboy looks like in his authentic regalia.

My wife thought I was a bit daft as I put my plan together. Grace even threatened to take a different seat on the plane should I get too carried away. Little did she know that I had booked the flight via London just to show off to whoever cared to feast their eyes upon this western Canadian-type cowboy.

As we planned and arranged to leave for Holland in May, I could hardly wait to don my newly acquired duds--cowboy boots, jeans, an open shirt with shining buttons, a denim jacket and

Because the majority of passengers on board from Western Canada were familiar with my kind, I was not too conspicuous boarding our first flight from Edmonton. It wasn't until we arrived in Toronto that I got a few second looks and sideways glances. In Montreal I got more extensive scrutiny. I could tell by their raised eyebrows how much they appreciated seeing a real live cowboy!

Arriving at Heathrow Airport safe and sound in London, England, we went to the waiting area to catch our flight to Amsterdam. It was there that I discovered more admirers. Several people gave me a once-over while a few teen-age girls walked by peeking and giggling: impressed, no doubt. Still, I felt a need for more exposure. I decided to visit the airport bar where the locals hung out.

I sat down beside a refined looking gentleman wearing a bowler hat. He was reading a magazine as I politely greeted him with my best "Howdy, Sir." He nodded but paid no further attention to me. I tried to tempt him with an offer to buy him a whisky on the rocks. Didn't work. He flipped a page on his magazine and angled his body so I was no longer in his line of vision. Oh well, so much for my attempt at cowboy camaraderie.

It was soon time to board our flight to Amsterdam. I tried to behave myself on the flight, much to Grace's delight. As we disembarked on the tarmac I spotted my parents watching from the second floor balcony. They did not indicate that they recognized us.

After going through customs, we climbed the stairs to where they were still standing. I stood right behind them, grinning, and asked who they were looking for. My elderly mother turned and gasped.

"Is that you, my boy?" "Yes, Mum," I answered and we embraced as if I were her prodigal son.

A week later we had a wonderful time celebrating my parent's anniversary in the village pub. We had dinner followed by speeches and a few poetry readings. I wore my cowboy attire again for the occasion. My contribution was to sing a variety of toe-tapping cowboy melodies. My musical contribution was well received. One uncle, who had visited Canada the year before, drank in the songs. His jaw dropped as he watched his crazy nephew blast out a few verses of Home, Home on the Range. After the festivities ended inside, we went outside and sat on the patio and enjoyed a short concert by the village music corps, to honor my parents' wedding anniversary. It wasn`t quite cowboy music, but it was entertaining nonetheless. I felt so intoxicated by the music that I emptied my glass of wine in short order. Then, in casual cowboy style (at least according to the movies) I threw my empty glass in a flowerbed beside me. Later, I was surprised to hear that a rumor was circulating about that goofy Canadian who had lost his manners! Oh Give me a Home Where the Buffalo Roam…

Horsing Around

1949: the summer season ended on my uncle's farm in Houston B.C.

I was looking for a new adventure. That is exactly what I got. I was assigned to take two horses to the lumber mill camp. These two horses had been roaming free during the summer on crown land. They had been lassoed by someone to be transported to the bush camp and used as skid horses.

I was used to working with horses and thought bringing these horses to the bush camp was a piece of cake. They appeared tame enough. One horse was quite big and heavy, a real draft horse, but easy to lead. The other horse was friskier but I considered myself a competent horseman and felt the best approach would be to ride the fat one bareback and lead the other horse by a rope on his halter.

The frisky horse, however, was much more spirited and had a temperament not unlike my own: "Don't tell me where to go." Both horses had been free all summer and were in no mood to be put back to work. All went well for a mile or two riding on a narrow gravel road and humming a song, "O what a beautiful morning!" Suddenly the two horses, sensing they were going in the wrong direction and away from the open range, stopped.

No urging helped; they would not move on. I slid off my horse and walked in front of them, holding the rope but they would not follow.

No way to get them to move with eight miles to go.

I tried subterfuge. Turning them around, I backtracked a few meters; then turned them around again. They would go for a few meters and stop again. I tried the trick once more, to no avail. They were smart; I needed to do something different.

I had no bridle for the friskier horse. Otherwise I would have ridden him and slammed my heels into his sides to make him move. When I thought I had a solution--tying the two of them together--the rope slipped out of my hand and the frisky horse (now named an S.O.B.) took off, trotting towards to the open range.

Quickly, I jumped on the fat horse again and pursued him. I realized that this clumsy horse could not keep up. It seemed hopeless. Just then a car came my way.

The driver saw the situation, stopped, and parked his car at an angle on the road. He got out of his car, spreads his arms wide and was able to grab the rope dangling from the horse's halter. I was greatly relieved. I'd had visions of pursuing that horse 10 miles or more in the opposite direction.

This time I tied the two horses' halters together. Then I cut a branch from a nearby tree. With enough rope to walk closely behind them and dangling the branch with its rustling leaves over their backsides I kept them at a brisk walk.

We stopped at a river crossing and I let the horses drink. We still had five miles to go.

We arrived at the bush camp in mid afternoon. I stabled the horses and, even though I didn't think they deserved it, gave them a big fork load of hay.

The fellows at the campsite laughed and joked about my ordeal, but knew I had earned their respect by getting the job done.

A few days later I was assigned to skid logs from the hilly forest to the sawmill. I had chosen the frisky horse, now my friend, to assist me. This horse gave me no more trouble. He liked me; I did not work him hard. I now named him Anthony (deserving praise).

He and I enjoyed the work: this horse and I had mutual respect for each other and were at peace. In the morning when I came to the stable he would neigh and put his snout on my shoulder as if to say, "I am ready for the day, if you are."

Language Skills

My brother-in-law Jan, 20 years my senior, and I boarded the train in Amsterdam on our way to Paris. Our train made a stop in Brussels, Belgium. A French woman boarded and took a seat in our compartment. I greeted her with "Bonjour, Madame."

Bingo, I thought when she responded. She understands the French I studied before leaving Canada.

This was the first time I had tried out my linguistic skills. To follow my greeting, I formulated a snappy, short French sentence in my mind. When I spoke it, I thought it perfect because she answered with a flood of wonderful French words. I understood nothing, however, except for her repeated phrase, "Mon Dieu." This was my baptism into the French language and, although I felt a little discouraged, I was not about to give up.

After changing trains in Paris we traveled on to Tours and were glad to soon settle into a cozy hotel. After supper I went for a walk. Jan had had enough for one day so he chose to stay behind and rest awhile.

As I strolled down the quaint streets of Tours, a thought struck me: France is known for a particular kind of liquor called Pernod, a greenish type of drink favoured by the fictional Belgium detective Poirot. My curiosity was piqued so I headed for a bistro a few blocks from our hotel. Entering this particular café-bar, I was welcomed by the owner with the usual greeting, "Bonjour, Monsieur. Vous désirez?"

I answered with my practiced, "Donne-moi un Pernod, s'il vous plaît."

It seemed I had found my French tongue; my linguistic training had not left me after all. The barman filled a medium-sized glass with Pernod liqueur and handed it to me.

"Voila, Monsieur."

Good, I thought, he understands me perfectly; maybe we can have some conversation and I can learn about some of the local culture.

The downed Pernod did its work: I was very relaxed. The bar owner asked if I played checkers. "Pas vraiment," I replied. I really was not sure of the rules.

"Il est très simple," he said, putting the checker board onto the bar. He set up a row of checkers across the board with a single check on the opposite side. His approach was to penetrate my single line of defense. He made three attempts and lost. Then he suggested we try one more time and bet me a whisky. I was confident that I could win and agreed, but in no time flat he broke through my defense and I lost the bet. Fait accompli, as the French say.

When I questioned him about the bill, which I thought seemed a bit high, he replied without hesitation, "Deux whisky!" It seems I had bought him a double shot along with my Pernod. Who was I to question the local establishment? Chalk it up to a French cultural experience.

As I looked at my empty Pernod glass my eyes moved to a bottle of white wine sitting on the counter. When the bartender saw me eyeing the bottle, he instructed his assistant to keep filling my wine glass.

The bar owner took his double whisky to a nearby table to play a card game. Of course, I needed to get full value after paying for his drink. I stuck around for an hour and managed to empty that bottle of Vin de Pays.

By the end of my stay, I was bordering on intoxication. After leaving the premises, I high-stepped down the street and exaggerated my own tipsiness. Music played in my head and joyful songs resonated on my lips, "As I was a walking one morning for pleasure, I spied this cowboy riding alone…"

I had not paid much attention to how far I had wandered. Eventually, I realized I was lost. Much to my chagrin, I knew the only way out of my predicament was to ask for help. I spied a woman and approached her. Our stilted conversation was getting me into more trouble.

Zut, alors!

OK, here we go: "Mademoiselle from Amsterdam…"

"Amsterdam?"

"Leon?"

"Armetier."

"Where is my bloody hotel?"

At that moment I bumped and staggered into Jan, of all people. He carefully led me to our hotel. Apparently he thought something was amiss when I did not return from my walk and decided to go looking for me. Likely my rendition of cowboy songs clued him in to my whereabouts.

It didn't take me long to get comfortable once Jan escorted me back to the right hotel. As soon as my head hit the pillow I was out. I found out later that my snoring kept my dear brother-in-law and protector awake for a quite a few hours, poor fellow. I, on the other hand, had a most restful sleep. We won't mention the throbbing temples the next morning!

Grand Prairie, AB

Dear Grace,

I am so sorry about not being able to see you this weekend. The rain is so bad, the roads are almost impassable. There is no way to travel by car or truck.

I miss you so much. I always feel so comfortable talking to you, as if I am at home with my own family--knowing and understanding each other, having a similar background, nothing to hide in our past, just feeling free and wanting to be together and hoping some day to be able to get together every day.

Living in a hotel for weeks on end gets so dull when rain prevents you from traveling and visiting farmers to discuss the value of their harvest. About the only thing that one can do is go to the bar for a beer, but you can only take in so much of that before it becomes boring too.

The days here, buying grass and clover seed for Steele Briggs Seeds, will end when the snow comes down in a week or two. Then I will be stationed in Edmonton, maybe until next summer.

Again, Grace, may I call you sweetheart? I am feeling so in love with you. I intend to buy a ring for you and hope and pray you will accept it.

Looking forward seeing you next week. In the meantime...

An ocean of love and, on every wave, a kiss.

Francis

Going Out for Dinner

It was the day of our 54th wedding anniversary: "Let's eat out, Francis," suggested my wife, Grace, "We should celebrate our 54th wedding anniversary. After all these years, we are still in love with each other so we should go out. Don't you agree?"

I had not thought of it. What was wrong, I wondered, with the dinner they serve here in our retirement home every day? "I'd just rather not eat dinner here to celebrate this special occasion," continued Grace, "and I am getting tired of the food here. It would be nice to eat out somewhere, just the two of us, and have time to talk and think about our past. What do you think, Francis?" It didn't take long to convince me and I happily agreed to the idea. The question was: where would we go?

"Well, you know dinner places better than I do," said Grace. "You decide, and make sure it's a nice place. You know I am a fussy woman when it comes to food, so find a nice cozy place."

I thought about the restaurant called Earls. I used to favour Earls many years ago, a restaurant that served my favorite clam chowder and pan bread with a beer on the side. Having stopped there the odd time when Grace went shopping with her woman friends, I had to look out for myself. Before leaving home, Gracie said that she was leaving her purse at home. "Yes dear, no problem. It's my treat," I agreed. So off we went on the day of our 54th wedding anniversary: February 17th, 2010.

We left early, before the restaurant would get too busy, so that we could take our time. We arrived there at 5:30 pm. There were very few customers at this early hour; the waitress gave us a lot of attention. Several menus were presented and we took time to study them for our preferences. I chose the wild salmon: my favorite. Gracie's choice was sirloin minion.

Before we had received our menus we had already shared a beer. Gracie thought it was over-doing it since we were also having a glass of wine with our dinner, but I asserted that we needed to relax and enjoy our time while we were there.

Although we had been at this restaurant before with friends, it had been a long time ago. Since retirement, we rarely ate out. Grace is such good cook and enjoys cooking, and we are fairly frugal about eating out.

When dinner was served, it looked very attractive with some fancy colored vegetables. Gracie ordered her favorite Merlot from the Napa Valley. We had stopped at a few wineries while driving though California one day many years previously and had tasted different wines in the Napa valley. We found that their Merlot was an excellent wine to go with her sirloin. At home we drink an African wine, an inexpensive wine called Roodeberg, which is also very satisfying.

I chose a chilled Sauvignon Blanc to go with my salmon. Both wines were within our budget and delicious, and gave our faces a shine. In the meantime, the restaurant was filling up, so we looked around and watched other guests between taking a bite of food or a sip of wine. All of the restaurant clientele appeared to be in as fine spirits as we were this evening.

When it was finally time to go home, I asked the server for our bill. Upon delivery, I was surprised to see it was for more than I expected. Oh well, we had had a good time and had enjoyed the meal, so I added a generous amount for service and signaled the waiter. Sticking my hand in my pocket to reach for my wallet, however, I found it missing.

I figured I must have put it in a different pocket, but no: no wallet there either. I looked at Grace and asked if she had her wallet. "No," she said, "Don't tell me you have no money."

"I must have left it on our dinner table at home," I said sheepishly.

"I told you I was leaving my purse at home and you promised to pay for the dinner," she scolded, "so now what? What will they do to us? Call the police?"

"No, we just have to be honest and tell them that we are sorry and that we will go and get it," I protested. We called the waitress and explained our problem. She called the manager. Grace's face changed color and she felt ashamed.

It did not take long before two people came over to see who we were, with half smiles on their faces. I explained who we were and that, no, I didn't have a driver's license or a certificate with our address with us. I told the manager that I would be happy to go home and get my wallet while he kept Grace here within eye-shot. The manager looked us over and studied our faces, then took down our names, address and phone number. He asked us to phone them with our Visa card number when we got home. "By the way," the manager asked, "do you happen to be the author of the book called *Journal of a Dutch Immigrant?*"

I nodded in the affirmative, and he told me that he'd read my book and found it very entertaining. His smile broadened as he said, "You sure did a lot of traveling and had some interesting encounters. Consider this one just another of your adventures!"

Grace and I left happy, although I did get some more scolding from my dear wife. At home, I discovered that my wallet was in my jacket, not in my pant pockets. I promptly phoned the restaurant and our dinner adventure was complete!

Kayaking

I watched someone paddling a kayak one day and it seemed easy. I was a good swimmer. In my younger days I had a canoe and enjoyed splashing around the neighborhood in small water channels in North Holland. I decided to take a few lessons.

For a number of years already, at the William A. Switzer Provincial Park, I had taken lessons to improve my skills in various other outdoor activities such as backpacking, hiking, and wilderness survival. I enjoyed those lessons and made use of my skills at every opportunity, hiking in the mountains.

Kayaking lessons were advertised in the newspaper. I was ready to take it on. Arriving at my first lesson, I met several skilled fellows ready to teach a bunch of us how to use the kayak. The lesson started with a lecture and I was not listening very well at first. After all, I figured, I was good at canoeing and kayaking couldn't be much different. After the lecture we got into the kayaks and were showed how to use the paddles. "Yeah, yeah," I thought, "I know all that."

Later, we were all directed to a 50 meter long swimming pool. Several kayaks floated there ready for our lessons which began with how to keep your kayak level and how to keep it straight: so far, so good.

The next lesson was how to keep your kayak from tipping and how to upright yourself if it did. Suddenly, I was less confident and staying level became very tricky. It required a lot of skill. A kayak is somewhat unstable and, once you lose your balance and don't have your paddle in the right position, you are in trouble.

The idea is to use your paddle to get yourself upright again and, if you are not able to do that, you will need to slip onto the spray deck or skirt over the cover that is attached to the rim of your kayak and swim. You'd have to try to rescue your kayak or swim for the shore if land is within your reach. Over and over we practiced trying to roll ourselves back upright by using a special paddle stroke. After each lesson, I came home totally worn out and realized that kayaking is definitely not a piece of cake.

After finishing the first course in Edmonton, I took a weekend off to go to William Switzer Provincial Park, north of Hinton where I met with a group of kayaking enthusiasts who planned to take on some wild rivers. After two days of practice in the park, our kayaks were taken to Whirlpool River south of Jasper which drains into the Athabasca River.

There we unloaded the kayaks and put them alongside the river. When all was ready we got into our boats and were given instructions on how to maneuver in the river whitewater. While it was mid-summer and the waves were only moderately high, it was plenty challenging for me. My first try to keep upright in the water was very short-lived. The waves managed to take me under; however, I managed to roll back upright in one successful swipe. The next try was not any better. I tried one more time when our supervisor saw me struggling and called me in to shore. Exhausted, I readily complied.

The supervisor then asked me if I would be so kind as to drive his truck to the place where all the kayakers would finish the course. I knew he was concerned that I would not be able to reach the destination we were heading for via kayak. Although I felt somewhat devastated, I accepted that it was probably for the best and agreed. So much for this tough fellow! I had to accept that my big dream of being a kayaker would not come to be. But, perhaps, this was understandable for one who had passed the age of fifty.

All was not lost, however, as a friend of mine had introduced me to canoeing. In 1982, Henry and I and four others canoed the Coppermine River. We headed to the Arctic coast from Lac La Grass (a hundred miles north of Yellowknife) to the Coppermine townsite at the Arctic Coast: 400 hundred miles over four weeks. It was the adventure of a lifetime!!

New Life

One particular Sunday morning, our Pastor delivered a sermon entitled: Did You See God's Leading?

That jolted me to attention. He used the analysis of Jacobs' son, Joseph, who was sold to a slave trader by his jealous brothers. He then ended up in Egypt, becoming the Administrator of that Kingdom. God put him there to look after his chosen people.

I did not think I had been led anywhere in my own life that I had not wanted to go. Then I wondered, really? I thought again, and realized: no, not to Egypt, but much has transpired in my life that wasn't really of my own choosing.

My parents taught my siblings and I, through Bible reading and especially by example, what it takes to live a Christian lifestyle. I became a strong believer too, but I wasn't really conscious of being led by the Spirit. I tended to follow the rules and the crowd: attending Church services and saying my daily prayers. My lifestyle was one of honesty and I tried to live the biblical call to "love your neighbour as yourself." I was not terribly good at loving my neighbour for too often I thought of myself, while not holier, still somehow at a higher level.

On reflection, however, I was astonished that the Spirit did lead me. I was simply not conscious of it. God has a way of using our sinful characters to His purpose. We think we are smart but God uses our weaknesses to get us go in His direction. We have a tendency to do and want, without asking God if it is good for us. I know God loves me and I believe He put a spoke in my wheels more than once, and, in hindsight, I am thankful.

Thinking back on my experiences over the years, I know I needed to listen more to what the Spirit was gently telling me. The evil spirit had a way of suggesting that I follow my selfish desires, but I see now how God employed a number of tactics to prevent His child from going the wrong way. For that I am forever grateful.

I can give thanks for even the difficult times in my life that, in the long run, were a blessing for me.

I have since learned to pray and to ask God what He has in store for me.

"Dear Lord, lead me. I want to be your servant!" is the prayer most often on my lips these days.

I am glad I did not have to undergo what Joseph went through, and I do not envy Joseph for his position in Egypt. What a responsibility! I did make my own journey, however, and, whether I always knew it or not, I was led indeed.

"Therefore, Lord God, thank you for giving me this new life, with Jesus as my Savior and the Spirit as my guide!"

Impatience

All my life I have been a restless person. I have to be on the move, see action or plan action. I've been happiest when taking on something new like a volunteer assignment, planning a vacation or changing my vocation. I was even involved in athletics.

I did well in long distance running. In 1972 I spent a great deal of time pursuing running as a sport. I ran a mile in 5 minutes and a 26-mile (42 KM) marathon in 3 hours which is equivalent to a 7-minute-mile average. That year my work performance suffered by about 40 % and so did my income, but it was fun in the meantime.

Impatience hampers careful planning. Even as I write this story my mind races ahead of my pen and I forget to think about grammar or how to construct the next thought. This, of course, results in having to re-write or missing an interesting detail.

Traffic tickets: many of them, I admit, are another result of my impatience. Speeding is a bad habit but difficult to control when driving a car with a 4 liter engine under the hood on a beautiful stretch of highway. Suddenly red lights are in your path: Oh no, not again!

Once, when I bought a new car, I was again reminded of my impatience. Whenever my car needed warranty repairs I was always given priority service without having to make an appointment. After several instances of jumping the queue, it became obvious that this would not last: one day I approached the service desk at the dealership without an appointment as usual. I strode in--insistence and annoyance clear in my body language. The shop foreman looked up from his desk and, seeing me, turned around and hollered to the mechanics, "Everybody stop what you are doing. Francis is here!" Well, I had a good laugh. I needed that message.

Impatience has caused me other embarrassments. In the past, while waiting in my car for my wife and children to join me to go for a drive, I'd grow so impatient and beep the car horn. Afterwards, I'd apologize but the damage was done.

Some years later I had a bicycle accident, which resulted in my becoming a left below-the-knee amputee. I couldn't drive and was dependent on my wife, Grace, for transportation. In the early months I used crutches and was slow getting from the house to the car. On a few occasions, in fun, Grace would beep the horn just to let me know how it feels to have the shoe on the other foot. I laughed about it. I had it coming!

Restless energy can be an advantage. Whenever a problem arose in the past, whether there was aggravation due to a repair job around the house or a communication breakdown between myself and another person, for example, I would deal with it right away. Fix what is broken, clear up misunderstandings or apologize immediately. This way, my mind was clear to move on to the other things on my agenda.

Impatience can also be an attribute. I experienced it in my sales career as a life insurance salesman. When making a presentation to a prospective customer, my body language tended to signal a subtle message of urgency and importance. It worked well for me: I became successful in my career.

My mother, many years ago, used to instruct me about being patient. She would say, "Francis, just watch the cat. It will sit hunched for hours to catch its prey." I don't know that I learned that lesson very well!

Mount Edith Cavell

I was on my way to Houston B.C. for a family reunion when I thought about re-visiting Mount Edith Cavell. I had visited there a number of times while back-packing in my younger years. I recalled, however, that when one arrives at the Jasper Park checkpoint they ask you, "Are you going straight through Jasper without stopping?"

Since they charge a bundle of cash I wondered if I might be given permission to make to make one short stop at this most attractive mountain. I decided to give it a try.

I arrived at the checkpoint where I stopped at one of the cubicles and was questioned by a striking woman with aquiline features and sparkling green eyes. She asked me where I was going and if I was going straight through without stopping. I answered, "I would love to take a short side trip to have a quick peek of my favorite mountain."

She asked, "What mountain? And what are your plans?"

I replied, "Oh, just to take a peek of Mount Edith Cavell to take a picture and then I'll be on my way."

"No," she said, "Besides, there is another checkpoint on the way." And with that, she was ready to dismiss me without mentioning, "You need to pay so much money to make a stop-over."

It gave me an idea. I took note of her French accent and started to twist my face into an anguished display of misery and stuttered, "Je me suis tres desole, Madam." Then I started to reach for my handkerchief while managing to shed a few tears.

Continuing to stutter, I wailed, "Il'ya une amputee extraordinaire. Je suis tres sorry. Thirty years ago I used to go hiking on those trails. Now I am an amputee and cannot walk anymore. S'il vous plait, Madam. Donne-moi a petite ticket for me to see Le Mountain for a few minutes to take a picture of Le Mountain for me to admire Le Mountain before I die?"

Madam looked at me with suspicious eyes and hesitated, but as I was still drying my tears she gave in and printed something for me to stick to my front window.

My face started to come back to a normal color and I wanted to voice my appreciation so I said, "Mercy bien, Madam. Vous etes a tres nice person."

After some more sweet adjectives, she waved me on and told me to get out of the way of the other travelers who were waiting behind me.

I continued on to Jasper and took a left turn onto Highway 93 going south and came to the next checkpoint. I was a bit concerned and wondered about having to answer more questions.

I opened the side window but did not say anything.

The serious looking woman just took a peek at the ticket on my window and said, "Bonjour, and have a nice day." I felt relieved and carried on to Mount Edith Cavell along the five mile, twisted, rough, and upwardly-steep road.

Meeting several cars and SUV's, I was surprised: I had never seen this much traffic thirty years ago.

When I reached the point where the mountain became visible there were so many vehicles. Not only was the parking area chuck-full, but cars were parked for a hundred meters along the road. I was not even able to park close enough to get out of my vehicle to take a picture!

Extremely disappointed, I simply stopped the car, grabbed my camera, opened the door, and shot a picture.

Only the very top of the mountain was visible.

I drove back to Jasper with a sorrowful feeling. Then again, I felt good that I got to see the mountain without having to pay any admission!

Pea Soup

Leaving home for work one morning, Grace said to me, "I am going to make your favorite pea soup today. You know: cook a pork hock; let it simmer; and, when ready, throw in one of those garlic sausages."

"Great going dear, I look forward to it. I'll be sure to be on time for supper!"

Later that afternoon, when the office was closing, two fellow office workers suggested we have a drink at the hotel across the street. Great idea, I thought and I joined them at the hotel bar. I ordered my favorite: vodka on the rocks.

While we chatted away, I noticed a young woman alone at the next table. She seemed somewhat forlorn, but I returned to face my friends. Then, taking another look a minute later and showing more curiosity, she smiled at me.

My compatriots wondered what was distracting me and looked behind them. I told them, "This lone woman is having a drink all by herself. Should we ask her to join us?"

"No," they replied. "We've got to go home."

"Me too, I guess, because Grace is making some special pea soup."

"Good for you," they said. "See you tomorrow."

I made a mistake taking a third look at the woman at the next table: she gave me a bigger smile. That did it. I had to investigate: Who is she and where is she from? Plainly, I was a bit nosy.

Over I went and asked if she would like some company. "Yes, by all means. You fellows seemed to have a good time together and I was envious of your camaraderie."

"Yes, we get along real well. What about you? Where are you from?"

"Oh, I am from Vancouver and needed a break."

"A break from your work?"

"No, I had surgery and my boyfriend was not very supportive. As a matter of fact, he met another woman while I was in the hospital for surgery."

"How did you find out?"

"Oh, he could not get it up when I returned from the hospital."

I thought to myself: Why is she telling me this? I was not used to such frank talk from a young woman. In the meantime, I ordered another drink and put the pea soup to the back of my mind.

After some more dialogue I asked her about her parents: where they lived, did they know where she was—that kind of thing.

"Not really," she replied. "They live in Ontario and don't care much about me." She then faced me, moving a bit closer to accentuate her cleavage and, smiling, said, "You are a good listener."

Yes, I thought, but where am I going with this conversation, and what is she seeking in me, or perhaps, from me? Not pea soup I'm sure.

She mentioned that she had a room in the hotel. Oh my! I am sure it would be nice to continue our conversation in her room.

I must break away, but how?

I started feeling sorry for her. I did not want to awaken my libido from hibernation, however. There were a few other people at the next table observing me, probably wondering if I would take the bait.

Fortunately, the image of the pea soup came back into view and broke my hesitation of whether to depart or not.

I suggested she call her Dad to tell him she loved him and that she would like to come home to visit. And, also, to let him know that she was broke.

Pea Soup! A powerful image, yes! Pea soup kept me in line, together with a picture of three smiling youngsters and a loving wife who trusts her husband.

The Country Southwest of Calgary

My wife Grace and I traveled to Calgary, and stayed there overnight with Grace's sister, Sherry. Grace wanted to go shoping with her sister for a day and I decided to revisit some beautiful country where, beside ranchers and farmers, bear and cougar have their habitat.

Since I had become an amputee in 1987, I had had dreams of camping and decided to do so in the foothills of Alberta which is incredibly beautiful.

I traveled from Calgary west on Highway #8 then south on #22 to Bragg Creek, thence west again on #66 to Elbow Falls all the while enjoying the scenery of forested hills with many campgrounds which I investigated for a possible overnight stay. Since it was still before noon, I thought to return later to make suitable choice. I wanted to visit the "Bar U" Ranch first, some 60 KM further south.

This whole route going south on # 22 and side roads going west you witness the beautiful green pastures and wooded hills as far as the eye can see. Beyond that you make out the majestic snowcapped Kananaskis mountains.

The highlight was to view the Historical "Bar U" Ranch that was started in 1880 by a rich family from eastern Canada. They leased this land (157000 acres or 63000 hectares) from the Canadian government. This place is just south of Longview. In 1890 they had over 10000 head of cattle and over 800 horses on their property. The cattle were raised for meat and the horses for racing and as workhorses. Later this ranch was divided into 6 smaller ranches and in 1991 a small parcel of 140 hectares became a historical place of interest where you can still view the old ranch house and other buildings.

You can get a guided tour riding on a historical hayrack pulled by a pair of gleaming black horses. The smell of leather on the harnesses caused me to revisit an earlier time when I first came to Canada in 1948. I had worked at that time with an identical hayrack and two horses for my uncle on a small ranch in mixed farming of grains and hay.

"Why was I camping in a tent by myself?" you might ask. It was nostalgia!

To my friends who asked the question: "Why are you going camping by yourself; such a lonely undertaking?" my answer was: "I intend to meditate."

I thought it would be good to be alone and think about my past and have some spiritual meditation in the process. They thought I intended to read the Bible and pray all day, but that was not what I had in mind. It was more about wanting to re-experience the glory of God's creation; viewing his handiwork in the foothills of Alberta with the mountains in the background. It has such a splendid vista you cannot help but praise God for the wonders He created!

Turkish Bath

(May 2001: touring 'The Silk Route' by train. From China to St Petersburg, one of our stops was in Bukhara, Uzbekistan.)

After a few days of sightseeing in the ancient city of Bukhara we had an afternoon to ourselves, so I pondered: what to do? Earlier in the day, on a walk about town, I had taken notice of a very old building made out of basalt stones: a Turkish bathhouse offering massages.

That was just what I needed!

I went on my own, dressed in a pair of shorts and wearing the peg leg that I use for taking showers instead of my normal prosthetic leg. In that attire, sporting my Tilley hat as well, I looked somewhat off-beat.

I rented a taxi for $2.00. The taxi driver dropped me off close to the building and I walked the rest of the way.

Upon entering the bathhouse, I was directed to the clothes lockers. While I undressed, I realized I had forgotten to bring a towel or an extra pair of under shorts. So there I was: buck naked!

The masseur lent me a thin, worn out towel and led me through a tunnel passage which had a low ceiling. The stone surface I was walking on was very slippery and I held on to my masseur for dear life, fearing I would fall or perhaps hit my head on the ceiling.

Entering the steam room, my masseur pointed to a spot where I was to lay down on my flimsy towel on a now extremely hot, flat, stone floor.

A roaring fire beneath the floor kept the stones very hot. A fellow traveler from France and I were lying there sizzling and cooking while wondering when the masseur would show up to give us our massages. We were sweating like horses after they had run in a heat wave.

After about fifteen minutes, the masseur signaled for us to rise from that inferno. He moved us to a different location where we could recover with a drink of water and to cool our bodies somewhat.

The masseur, a man of small stature, was ready to go to work. He had me lay on my back on this flat stone floor that was not quite so hot. He started to work on all my ligaments from head to toe. He did a good job massaging and pummeling all the body parts, until he reached my right arthritic knee. When he put pressure on it, I cried out, "Ouch!"

"Problem?" he said: one of the few words he knew in English.

"Yes," I replied.

He let up on the knee and continued to other body parts until he got to the other knee and asked again, "Problem?"

I answered "No."

He finished with the front and had me roll over onto my belly; still on that measly, thin towel. Lying face down, he worked me over: starting with my shoulders, down my arms, pummeling my bum and down my legs. Now and then he questioned me: "Problem?"

"No. No problem."

When he was almost finished, he touched my back followed by the refrain, "Problem?"

Thinking he was asking if I had back problems, I replied, "No."

Before I knew what was happening, my masseur started walking all over my back. Although he was a short person, he still weighed about 130 lbs and all I could do was gasp for air. I was unable to cry out, "Yes, problem!"

Fortunately he did not take a long walk and I felt relieved when he came down from my then-tender body. His last words were, "You fini!"

I took a few deep breaths and wondered if my spine was still in good order.

Stepping out the door, the thirty degree temperature seemed remarkably cool in comparison to the hot-house inside.

Young Man's Christian Association (YMCA)

I have lived so many years with so many blessings!

I came to Edmonton in 1952 from northern B.C. and, now and then, I visited the YMCA. Later, as an insurance agent, I became somewhat overweight and figured the YMCA might help me get back to physical fitness. So, in 1964, while living in the west end of the city, I started to visit the "Y" and became a regular for about 10 years. When we moved a significant distance away from the "Y" I took up track and field activities, as well as hiking and back-packing in the mountains.

In 1982 I went on a canoe trip to the Arctic coast from Lac la Grass in the N.W. Territory to the town of "Coppermine," a distance of 640 km which took four weeks. After that, I took up running. Over the years I ran several 42-kilometer marathons. When my legs began to give out, I took up cycling until someone with a pickup truck hit me from behind and I was catapulted into a ditch.

From there on in, I had to accept that I would be a left, below-knee amputee. After more than 2 years in recovery, I gradually moved from a wheelchair to a cane. I was happy to see the Jamie Platz YMCA being built, which was closer to our home in the west end of town. It was finished in 1989. I have been a member there ever since.

It has been a tremendous blessing for me! I was able to go swimming any day of the week. The swimming allowed me to exercise without pain or discomfort. It did not take long until I was able to swim a mile most days of the week. An additional enjoyment was meeting friendly people at the "Y", young and old persons with varying status in life.

The word Christian is hardly used but the staff does live up to the mission. For example, once when I hurt myself and was nearly in tears the manager took note and gave me a hug which lifted my spirits up. I went home with much gratitude and happy to be a member of the "Y."

Wrestling Match in Beijing, 2001

My friend Peter and I had arranged to take a tour called The Silk Route. This tour would start in Beijing and end up in St. Petersburg, Russia. The tour group would spend 10 days in China and make stops in Kazakhstan and Uzbekistan. Peter and I arrived in Beijing a few days ahead of the tour group. This gave us time to get acclimatized and to orientate ourselves before the rest of our group arrived.

The first day we did some sightseeing in the neighborhood of our hotel. The next day, straying a little further, we saw a restaurant advertising Peking duck. We decided to try it out. This restaurant was classier, having tables covered with linen cloths and napkins.

We both ordered the dumplings and Peking duck as advertised. When our plates of Peking duck arrived, we looked at them: the ducks were nicely arranged but their eyes were staring at us accusingly.

This display did diminish our appetites a little, but we managed to twist the ducks' necks to cover their now sad eyes. We still ate the ducks with less relish than we had first anticipated.

After a walk around the neighborhood my legs and feet were tired and getting sore.

We decided to take a rickshaw back to our hotel: those two wheel chariots pulled by quite muscular men. We approached them, and using mostly hand signals we were quoted 15 dollars for each rickshaw. To be sure Peter was quick to get confirmation and asked: "Chinese dollars?" (Meaning Chinese currency called Yuan) The driver nodded his head. There was room enough in the rickshaws for two but the man who had to pull the rickshaw had taken a look at us and seeing that we were 6 feet tall and weighed over two hundred pounds each, directed us to take separate rickshaws.

We hoisted ourselves into those, what I later called, 'Chariots, pulled by Spartacus.'

It was rather exciting being pulled along side streets and crossing a few intersections viewing other traffic. Our chariots' runners stopped a half a block away from the hotel entrance.

To be cautious, while my man pulled me along, I had peeled off 15 Yuan from a bundle of Chinese currency and put them in a separate pocket. I did not want my Spartacus to see the amount of money I carried. When we disembarked from our rickshaws, Peter pulled his money from his pocket and gave his man 20 Yuan. My leather-faced Spartacus saw what his cohort received and wanted the equal amount from me which I refused because we had agreed to 15 Yuan. He then grabbed me by the wrist. He was as strong as an ox. I grabbed his wrist, too, trying to wrestle free. No chance: he was 25 years younger and battle-hardened.

In the meantime, Peter had started to walk on ahead. I hollered at him but he did not return. I tried to scare my driver by threatening to call the police. He just laughed. I thought maybe I should just give him the extra 5 Yuan but was hesitant to do so.

I was loath to show the bundle of cash I carried. My next thought was to knee him in the crotch and then get away from him. I realized he could overtake me quicker than I could walk and I was unable to run due to wearing a prosthetic leg. Luckily, he finally gave up and let me go on my way. I heaved a sigh of relief and caught up with Peter at the hotel entrance with my bundle of cash still intact.

Signing books

Signing books is an interesting word for selling one's books. I liked that idea. Selling books may be a different word for selling your book, but people love to meet the author and I love to meet my readers. So here I go:

I saw a woman entering the Chapter's Bookstore. She was of medium height, and I guessed her age to be about 35. She had bright blond hair and dressed in a dark suit with a white blouse. I assumed her to be a person who had an office position.

I was sitting behind a small desk close to the bookstore entrance selling my books when I made eye contact with this well-dressed woman. She appeared to have no intention of stopping on her way to her intended place in the store. I was able to get her attention with my smile, however. I wore a three-color striped cotton shirt covered with a chain necklace and a summer cap embroidered with the name Aruba on it. I introduced myself as the author of the book on display called Journal of a Dutch Immigrant. She became curious and took a look, read the reviews, asked questions and said, "I am a writer myself. I write magazine articles." Then she left but came back 10 minutes later and bought a copy of my book.

In the meantime, another woman had heard some of the conversation about my book. She mentioned that she planned to make a trip to Holland to visit her friends. I suggested that my book would be a good one to read while traveling. After some hesitation she bought one. Then a few minutes later she came back and wanted a second copy for another friend in Holland. "Good going!" I thought. I was very happy how the sales were going.

Looking at the clock I realized that I had sold five copies of my book in the first hour. I smiled to all who entered the store and some, out of curiosity, would come closer. I let them hold a copy of the book while answering some of their questions. One gentleman dressed as a businessman was a chiropractor and was curious about selling books, since he also had written a book. Informing him how to go about it, I encouraged him as much as I could. He was happy that I brought it to his attention and also bought one of my books!

After four hours of meeting so many book lovers I had reached my objective of 18 sales for a particular day. I was as happy as a peacock in the summer. My never ceasing smiles faded and my lips resumed the normal position! I went home, had a cup of coffee followed by a class a wine, and then it was time for a nap on my comfy old, easy chair.

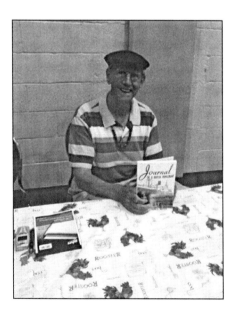

March 2010

On a later day visiting a different store, I met a woman who I believe was a teacher. She took look of my book and turned it over to read the preview on the back of my book. She looked at me and said, "You are a Christian." (She was reading the review where the text ended; that the author loves is God). She came closer and said. Can I give you a hug? I was perplexed but felt honored to have some one took note of me being a Christian, and gave her permission. She took the book and came closer, to give me a hug. Being moved by her words I kissed her cheek and dropped a tear. It made my day.

Signing books continued…

I arrived at Indigo one Saturday noon to sell my books and settled down at the pre-arranged table to display my books, "Journal of a Dutch Immigrant." Sitting behind the table I faced the entrance on my right and could keep an eye on the cash register on my left. I was happy with that arrangement, though I did not expect to sell many books since the previous time, a few months ago, sales had been poor.

I organized the books, putting some on the left side and others on the right side of the table, and displayed some on plastic stands to attract the eyes of customers. When I was ready, I raised my head and set my face in the sweetest way. Almost immediately an elderly couple came up and asked me if I was the author. When I replied yes, they told me that they too were born in Holland. With very little ado, they bought a copy. I was somewhat pleasantly perplexed with such a nice start in selling my books. Usually I have to get their attention by making a comment while they are passing me with averted eyes. These two Duchies drew another customer's attention that became curios and also bought a copy of my book. A few minutes later a young woman with a child holding came to my table, took a look on my book, read the title, and said: "Ik spreek ook Hollands" (I also speak Dutch) She was born in Canada, but her parents had taught her to speak Dutch when she was still a child. Of course, she needed a book for her parents living in the Peace River country. And so it went for a half hour, selling a book every 5 minutes.

I was still perplexed but naturally happy. I had only 14 books with me and they would be sold in two hours.

Well, not quite that fast...the traffic in the store had been just right at that moment. The next half hour I only sold two books. Just the same, I had never experienced that much interest. The next two hours were much slower again. I kept my eyes on shoppers who came through the entrance and also looked at the register so now and then, watching people paying for their books and wondering if I missed a possible customer. Once, I took note of a middle-aged person who bought a number of books, which almost filled his satchel. I was curious of what he bought and hoped he would look in my direction. Sure enough he turned my way, holding his load over his shoulder. Having eye contact, I asked if he had some space left. Seeing his surprised surprise look, I told him that I could help him fill his bag with one more book. He became curious, took a look, and said, "You are right, I have a friend from Dutch background.

I will buy one of your books. He went back to the cash register and paid for the book and waved to wish me success. Later, I talked with the woman who took his money, and asked her how much he spent. It was almost 175 dollars.

Sometime later, I met another person curious about my book and how I sold them. He was direct. He had watched me selling books, and was eager to have some conversation. I asked him to stay out of the way of potential customers who might come near, so he squatted beside the table. He was considerate enough not to want to interfere with me selling books. He was from Newfoundland but was employed in Alberta. We had an interesting conversation,

I liked his colloquial language, but I needed to keep my focus on my task at hand. He understood and left with a big smile.

Three hours passed and I had sold my 14 books. A week later, I had a conversation with a friend, a retired Pastor and author of a book about his background and family. He was a clever writer and often bested me in writing interesting stories and he is also good in delivering his stories to audiences. When I told him about my success in selling my books, he expressed surprise, because he had difficulty selling his books. Only a few sold in a particular day, he said. So I told him, "Well now my dear friend, you kept me on the straight and narrow from the pulpit. Now it is my turn to shine, to be the best seller of books. You can't have it all."

Later I became aware about Farmer Markets around Alberta, they will accept persons who wish to sign, or sell, books. So I went to find the best places to sell my books. Some farmer's markets in Edmonton are asking too much money within the city: markets where they sell all kind of products but mostly vegetables. I took advantage of that opportunity and most of my sales have been around places near Edmonton, my home. Finding places not too far from my home since the cost of fuel may take away one's profit.

Some of my customers are born in Holland as well, as I was. More often the second generation or third would buy a book for their parents who immigrated to Canada many years ago. Other consumers love to buy non-fiction books, buying my book for their parents or friends. Then we have persons who love to talk but are not interested in obtaining my book. Some have questions and love to talk, and are not interested buying my book. Then I ask them if they are interested in the book or just to talk?

At my age of 82 my memory has slowed down, at times I get stuck finding the right words and have difficulty answering their questions.

More about my condition of memory loss you will find in the last part of this book.

Selling books needs some skill and patience. My problem is: my patience is short, and I have to talk to myself, to relax and wait for a person loves my product. My mother at age 70 years was told me, Francis, "Just watch our cat who waits until she catches her rat." I never forgot that.

It was at a particular Saturday morning attending a farmer's market 150 kilometer away from our home in Edmonton. I was there by 9 o clock. So here I was ready in my chair watching for the public showing up at our market at 9.30 Am. It was waiting until the first people slowed up about 30 minuets later, and wondered if any one would show up, when slowly people crossed the street walking, or came by car. I took a big breath to be ready to get their attention. However most of the comers came here for fresh vegetables and they did not have eyes for this book signing. I felt disappointed, but my mother words came back to my mind. When more shoppers showed up and walked closer to my table, which I had set up so neatly with books, I was able to get their attention by using my system of smiling and nodding, holding a copy of my book and waving it a bit. Then gradually book lovers caught their attention and were taking a look, then asked a few questions and then became excited and quickly bought a copy of my book called "Journal of a Dutch Immigrant" holding them with eagerness and ready to read the stories.

And it turned out that thirteen books were sold, and I drove home with joy in my heart, meeting my beloved wife Gracie who had cooked a delicious meal. And of course the wine to go with it added a big smile.

Telegrapher (1953)

It was on my days that I became unemployed from a farmer not far from Edmonton. It was not my intention to go back to be employed there again. I had enjoyed the summer with the farmer, who was a kind person, and enjoyed my time at the farm.

I had taken this employment to get familiar with Edmonton, where I intended to find employment. In my past experience I was employed with a Wholesale Seed Company, which sells and buys up different types of seeds such as grass and vegetable seeds.

It was then that my brother in-law Henry suggested I try telegraphing since he was employed as a telegraph operator for the Canadian National Railway. I was not looking forward sitting on a chair. It was the last type of employment that I had in my mind. Then again, since Henry made me see that it might be an opportunity, he argued that I could handle that type of work. I thought about it and, since I was getting ready to get on my way to get on a train to Halifax to take a boat to visit my parents in Holland, I asked Henry for a book on the Morse codes to study while traveling before I would make a decision.

I returned six weeks later to Edmonton. I had studied and practiced the Morse code quite a bit, but was far away from being ready to apply for this difficult type of the Morse code language. In the meantime, Henry had contacted some of his telegraph friends about me having some interest to learn the system as a telegrapher. One friend who lived in Tofield was willing to take me to his home for several weeks to learn and practice to be a telegraph operator. It became the most difficult type of employment I ever experienced: hitting the buttons on a practice device, sometimes ready to throw it out of the window.

Only the inner voice kept me from doing so, and I would return to the practice set another day.

I finally did pass my exam and was employed by the CNR in April of 1953 as a telegraph operator and assistant station agent. I worked there until January 1954. This experience helped me to improve my vocabulary and grammar skills and my ability to deal with the public.

However, over time, and being stationed on different train stations within about 100 kilometers to Edmonton I had the responsibility of watching the telephone to receive orders to stop a train or to give the train a sign to carry on towards the next station. One particular day I wanted to take a ride with one of the trains that had stopped at our station to let another train pass by. I phoned the stationmaster in Edmonton and asked him if I could have leave and make use of the train which was on the way to Edmonton at 5 AM. Yes, that was OK and I closed the station and took off with the train to Edmonton. I forgot to change the signal for the next train that did not have to stop, however. This made the signal operator in Edmonton madder than a hoot-owl. They had to awaken another telegrapher, who lived above the station, to change the signal flag to let the train continue. While he talked to the Master Operator, he informed him that I was a bad operator. I was told not to return to the station where I was employed and was dismissed from that position. Instead, I was demoted to be cashier at another train station. It suited me fine. I received the same income as before. From there on in, I enjoyed my new position until some small train stations were not used anymore and I was not needed anymore.

From there I went to Steelbridge Seed Company, who where happy to accept me since I had previous experience at my father's seed company in the Netherlands. I stayed with that company for 5 years. Then someone came to see me and I was hired as a "Life Insurance Agent," which lasted 30 years until my retirement in 1987 when I became disabled when a car catapulted me into a ditch.

My Loved One

Her name is Grace: the woman whom I married in 1956. She is a graceful person and, often, I call her Gracie.

Grace has a lot of patience with her husband who is always in the way. She has to put up with me, her husband Francis, who loves to travel to places which she is not interested in. There is a definite "no" for places where language and types of food are not of her interest. But she always listens to me when I talk about the places I want to go to, even when she has no interest at all. She has difficulty making choices: instead of telling me where she wants to go she would say, "Why in world would I want to go there?"

Since we had three children over the span of seven years, it was difficult to leave our home together. In the meantime, I was often away from home due to my type of work. I left my Gracie at home with our three daughters all alone, although her brother John and his family lived across from our house.

In some ways Gracie missed her freedom and being able to meet friends at places away from home. There were times when she was not able to leave her children, except to go to the outhouse which was built onto the back of our home and to which, in winter time, you had to walk over some slippery snow. There was no running water in our home.

Once, Grace mentioned that she could not get away without having someone in to take care of her children. When I suggested that she could walk to the outhouse and have some fresh air, she got mad as hoot owl. Her eyes, always friendly, became so dark and scary. I realized that, even if I wanted to, I could not even get close enough to give her a kiss. I was taught something from this that was very important: from there on in, I learned to give more attention to my sweetheart.

Over time, I became a member of the YMCA: swimming and taking part in some excursions with other fellows. By then our three daughters were going to school and, when Grace saw her chance, she took lessons in swimming and other activities as well.

Grace also loved watching Oprah Winfrey on television which I thought was a foolish interest. Therefore, in order to fool me, my Gracie would hang up her bathing suit in the bathroom to make me think that she had gone to the YMCA for a swim.

Eventually, my goofy woman realized that Oprah was not that important and she decided to run with me. This exercise turned out badly since I was almost twice as fast as her.

It was then that Grace took up gymnastic exercises (walking 2 kilometers each way to the YMCA) She even made me take a picture which showed me that she was a can-do woman. She also impressed me greatly when she turned herself over on the floor. At that point I saw her as a tough woman: stay out my way, Francis, if you think you are the only one that is in good shape!

Many years later I lost my ability to run and can now only walk a short distance due to a person who drove his car into me while I was on my bike. After the accident, it took three years before I could walk without a cane or wheelchair. In the meantime, Gracie kept up her activity and still walks 3 kilometers three times a week.

I am a lucky fellow: having Gracie as my wife!

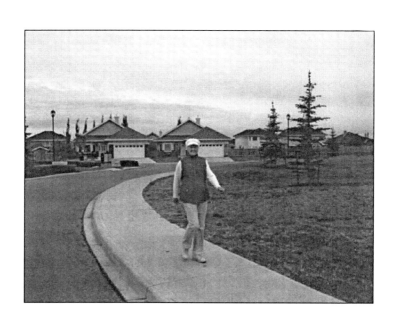

Maastricht, the Netherlands

We were invited to Andijk to celebrate a gathering of cousins within the Ruiter clan: the grandchildren of my parents, Gerrit and Lida Ruiter. When I received the invitation from my niece via e-mail, I became very excited about meeting all my nieces and nephews, my brother Piet (the last of my brothers) and my three sisters. I invited my three daughters to come along to meet their nephews and cousins as well.

I contacted Piet by e-mail and suggested that, while I was visiting, the two of us make a trip to Maastricht, a three-hour trip by train from Hoorn. Maastricht is the most southerly city of the Netherlands.

For me it was a place of history: about 2000 years ago, during the time of the Roman Empire, Maastricht was where the soldiers rested and prepared for further expansion of the Empire. Piet liked the idea of visiting this "Bourgonsische city" as well. He had visited Maastricht a few times before with his wife who passed away some years ago and, therefore, was a place of memories for him.

Pete and I got on the train and enjoyed the scenery along the way. We relaxed and talked about our past while taking in the view of towns and cities and several rivers; one of which was the Rhine that goes from Switzerland going through Germany, Rotterdam and at the North Sea.

Arriving in Maastricht around noon we took a taxi to the 100 year old hotel called Amrat du casque. The elevator was old fashioned but the beds were neat and soft, and the bathroom was spacious with a deep tub: large enough for me to stretch out my six-foot length. After eating lunch close by and dropping our overnight handbags in the hotel, we walked over to the city center which was just around the corner.

Piet and I climbed into an electric train on rubber tires which was ready to take us for a ride through town. The train was a small rusty electric one powered by electric batteries which got their energy from the sun shining on the steel roof.

The inner city was very old with a population of only 150,000. We moved slowly through the oldest part of the city on narrow streets competing with hundreds of visitors walking along the same streets. The driver gave constant commentary about the different buildings. Some of the churches were built several hundreds of years ago and are not used as much anymore as when they were first built. We also passed a Museum Cathedral: a special University that teaches language translation from Dutch to French, English or German for students who wish to be able to translate for businesses who need translated information of their products.

The street from our hotel towards the River Maas was full of visitors stopping here and there; shopping or having a snack. Now walking, Piet and I reached the River where we took a boat ride up and down the river for an hour. There wasn't much to see, but it kept us cool, and we enjoyed a beer and a snack while watching other guests.

Time moved on and we were ready for supper. Near our hotel again, we found a classy restaurant serving delicious meals. We sat at a separate table to rest our tired legs from all our walking. Studying the menu, we chose salmon together with several vegetables and, of course, a glass of white wine for additional taste to top off our happy outing.

Since it was noisy inside and the weather was still warm, we sat outside and watched the people going by. We talked more about our past and our present, sharing our thoughts about ourselves and how we see the world around us.

We also reflected on the differences between our countries: Canada and the Netherlands. Canada is so large with such vast distances and great variances in terrain, such as flat prairie and immense mountains--difficult to imagine or describe. The Netherlands, on the other hand, is so small and flat but very cozy.

In our youth--being close to school, having smaller stores, and everyone biking--we felt warmth. Even today there is no space for automobiles in the inner cities. You find hundreds of bicycles beside all train stations from where people walk or use a bus or ride a tram to get to their destinations in city centers.

I thoroughly enjoyed these few days with my brother Piet. In a sense, I had missed him since I was 16 years old when Piet was a soldier in Indonesia for several years. In the meantime, I had immigrated to Canada. After that I did not see him again for a number of years.

Back in our rooms, we prepared ourselves for the party of our 90 year old sister-in-law, Janny Lotteraman, at the Dorps Huis in Andijk. There, I would meet many more of our family and friends.

This first part of my outing in Holland was successful and rewarding.

Papa and Three Daughters

I invited my three married daughters to come along to The Netherlands where I was born, and they readily accepted. Their husbands encouraged them to go for it since I promised to pay for the trip. I did have an ulterior motive though. First of all, I had received an e-mail inviting all the cousins (grandchildren of my parents, Gerrit and Lida Ruiter) to come together in August of 2010. It was to be a reunion, something we'd done as siblings and extended families 20 years ago.

One of the cousins, my dear niece Truus, took it upon herself to send invitations to us and organize the set-up for this special day. I and my siblings and their spouses were not invited to the entire day's events, but were encouraged to attend the evening festivities and dinner. The cousins were invited to get re-acquainted with Andijk, where most of their fathers or mothers were born. They were given a map to find their way to different pre-arranged places of interest, using bicycles for transportation. The cyclists went to the homes where their parents were born and where their grandparents had lived. They cycled on top of the dijk (dike) overlooking a very large lake where steamboats, motorboats, and sailing boats showed their sails or steam pipes.

By five o' clock, we elderly people (mostly in our 80s) joined the younger generation who were already gathered together imbibing in various drinks with excited faces, getting to know their cousins who come from different parts of Holland and from Canada.

We Oma's and Opa's greeted our nieces and nephews with hugs and kisses: three times on the cheek--left, right and left again. I welcomed these enthusiastic and intimate greetings!

We sat around with our cousins at several different tables. From where I sat looking over the length of our table, I noticed someone waving in my direction. I did not know the person and paid no attention, but a few minutes later when I happened to gaze in that direction again, this same woman was waving once more. I decided to go and visit.

When I settled myself next to her, she hugged me and kissed me with great enthusiasm. I was at a loss, but very flattered. She then explained, using colloquial language, who she was and that she also came from the town of Andijk. More importantly, she told me that she had visited my wife and me in Canada quite few years ago while she was staying with a sister and two of her brothers who lived in Edmonton. Gradually my memory revived and, with my second drink, I gave her a hug as well: warming up to a good conversation.

The party continued with a delicious three-course dinner provided by Gerrit Ruiter, the president of Holland Select Seed Company in Andijk. Gerrit is named after his grandfather and it was his great-grandfather who started the company about hundred years ago. Gerrit travels around the world to sell his vegetable seeds to large growers.

There were a few musicians who led us into some familiar songs of many years ago. The party continued until about 9 PM when most of us older ones had enough and others had to travel to their own homes around the country.

Of course, my daughters' other interest was shopping. Fortunately, we stayed in a B&B close to my sister Caroline who lived in Canada some years ago but returned to Hoorn to take her former position as a nurse. She showed my daughters around the well-known city of Hoorn and its 400-year-old harbor. During the 17th and 18th centuries, ships traveled from this harbor to Indonesia loaded with costly spices that were sold to neighboring countries making Holland rich.

While my daughters walked around town, I parked myself at a hotel where I was told to stay put and not get lost. I had no trouble waiting for the shoppers while I indulged in a few Heineken beers.

One day, we took the train to Delft: a city I love to visit and where we also have relatives. It was a 764 year old city by this date in 2010. In the 16th century, the Spanish army occupied part of Holland. When the Spanish army attacked that city of Delft the people flooded the land around the city in order to prevent the Spaniards from overtaking them.

I had visited Delft a number of times since my wife had been born there. While visiting, we would often shop around the inner city and enjoy a lunch of salted herring or smoked eel. This time, however, my daughters called the shots. Before leaving Canada, their mother had given them express instructions to look after their Dad. My wife's concern was about my mobility and some cognitive impairment. So, after having lunch with relatives in Delft, a nephew drove us to the city center and deposited me at a restaurant called Stad's Coffee Huis where I was asked to stay until they returned from a brief shopping spree. Since it was a rainy day and my mobility was not up-to-snuff, and because they'd been warned to watch over me, I accepted their proposition. An as they left, however, I did walk for a few minutes within sight of the coffee house. Then I made myself comfortable on a chair near some other people drinking coffee or reading a newspaper. My choice was a Heineken beer, followed by a coffee and a cookie, while I patiently waited for my daughters to show up.

I had intended to show them the place where I bought the painting hanging in our home. Years ago, 1976, I purshased it near the city center. At that time, I remember, a bearded man was sitting on the stone entrance of the building which I intended to enter. I thought he was a street person, but when I went inside he followed me and made me aware that he was the artist.

I also wanted to show them the Fish Market where I would always stop to buy (and swallow) a salted herring. The city center has a large open weekly market. On one side is the City Hall facing a church built in the 17th century called New Church. A few streets away was the 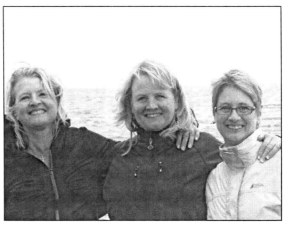 old church which was built in the 16th century. So interesting when in Canada a building of fifty years is considered old!

When the girls did show up we headed for the train station to return to our B&B in Hoorn. I do admit that I felt left alone in Delft, but I was happy for my dauthers who had a good time. I had experienced Delft many times before when I was in better shape.

It was a great day, and we began to prepare ourselves for returning home to Canada.

Taxi
1953: Single, Unemployed, and Running Out of Money

It came to me to apply for a position as a taxi driver. Even though I was not too familiar with the city, I was hired.

Arriving for duty at 8 am the following morning, I settled into my appointed car: # 29. The dispatcher called and directed me to an address near our office.

I found it readily, but I was still a bit nervous.

My first fare was a man with his pregnant wife who needed to go to the Misericordia Hospital. Uh oh: this did not bode well for me.

I knew the district in which the hospital was located, but not its exact address.

Dwelling on the problem of location, I suddenly came to the first set of stoplights. I stepped on the brakes too hard and heard a groan from the back seat. "Sorry Ma'am," I stammered. "The lights changed too quickly."

Phew. Thank goodness: no premature arrival.

I did find the hospital and asked the man if I should wait. "Not with you behind the wheel," he replied.

Sorry sir.

At least I now know where the hospital is located!

The following days I was assigned to a more delicate part of Edmonton. I was instructed to park in front of the hotels on 96 Street, between 101st and 103rd Avenues.

I was getting a new type of clientele too: mostly those who wanted transportation from one hotel to another hotel within a six-block area.

It seemed strange to me: requesting transportation within walking distance. Why not walk a few blocks?

Then a personal call came in for taxi number 29.

Now why would I get a personal call? Odd; really odd!

The call was from a woman who needed transportation from a downtown hotel to her home in north Edmonton. As I drove her home, she talked about a sailor she'd met who was not very experienced. I did not make the connection to her profession at first, but it came to me when she pulled out her wallet to pay for her fare and out spilled a condom.

I realized then that I was a greenhorn and needed to learn fast.

On another occasion, a call came through for taxi number 29 from a girl about eighteen years old. She was pretty and asked to be driven to a spot about four blocks away. She started to make conversation and giggled a bit then suggested we go somewhere and have some fun. I was lost as to what she meant. My brain cells worked overtime.

What does she mean? Am I a candidate about to be educated on how to have fun?

My hormones had not yet been educated as to what it meant to "have fun." They, in fact, were rudderless, you might say.

My brain, however, was catching on... I think.

My hormones must have finally had some indication as to direction: they were forming a battle troupe for possible action and waited for orders to go...where?

Finally, my hormones got wise to what was likely in the making. They moved into my loins, forming a ready battalion and waiting with great anticipation for the word: "Go for it!"

I felt my blood pressure rising and my face blushing when the allure of perfume entered my nostrils. My throat was getting dry.

The radio crackled.

"Calling number 29... Number 29, where are you?"

I took a deep breath.

"Sorry. Duty calls: no time to have fun."

I was saved to be a derelict to myself.

Side note: It wasn't until later that I learned that the previous driver of taxi number 29 had been a pimp!

The Great Plains

My son-in-law Phil and I traveled to Sioux Centre, South Dakota on June the 6th: meeting fellow enthusiastic sojourners at Dordt College. Forty, mostly seniors, men and women, were introduced to each other. Two couples were from Canada. The others came from within an area of a thousand miles.

We were introduced to our travel plans around Iowa, Minnesota and South Dakota. Traveling in a 50-seat brand-new bus, with Bill van Beek as our chauffer, we were amazed with his skill driving this large bus through narrow roads and farmers' gates and maneuvering in their back yards.

Dianne was in charge, organizing our travels and places to sleep.

James Schaap was our storyteller: mostly about the history of the Indian war with the settlers who had taken over much of the Indian Territory.

Robb De Haan, our biologist, lectured on the history of places we visited and explained how the landscape and soil became so fruitful.

We traveled through the wonderful rich country of Iowa, Minnesota and South Dakota. My wife Grace and I had traveled through this country on our way to Arizona once, escaping the winter in Canada. We had paid little attention to the landscape or crops. Our interest was to have a look at Dordt, and then continue on to our winter home in Apache Junction, Arizona. This time I felt ashamed as a person who lived in a horticulture area, where I was born, and whose father grew different kinds of vegetable crops. This time Robb got my full attention. He made us see the fruitful land, land that once was covered by ice and snow more than a billion years ago.

He explained how rocks traveled during the ice age in snow from the North (Canada), which gradually crushed the rocks into soil. At the present, Iowa and Minnesota grow mostly corn and other types of food products. I found the landscape and farmland very neat. It reminded me of Holland where you see similar neat landscapes.

This same land was once occupied by Native Americans, from 900 AD, and the population grew to 5000 Indian people at around 1500AD to 1725 AD.

Traveling towards Minnesota, we took note of about a thousand wind turbines in south west Minnesota: a new energy source which benefited some farmers with extra income; however most of the electricity is sent to the large city of Chicago.

Not every one is happy with the wind turbines; they have changed the landscape. We traveled on to our overnight stay at the Guardian Inn, in Windom, MLN.

Day Two:

The evening before we had a discussion concerning a small Lutheran Church that became too small to continue due to young people leaving the farm, moving away from home and finding employment elsewhere. Church attendance became very small. Consequently they had to sell their church. Many people where heart-broken. They made a movie about how they removed the church itself; transplanting it elsewhere.

Consequently some of the parishioners transferred their membership to the nearest Lutheran church. We visited that church to share our Christian faith by serving the same God. We were welcomed by the congregation and asked to stay for lunch in appreciation of our interest through their difficult time.

We continued on to the Jeffers Petroglyphs, a site preserved from the American Indians who lived there 8000 years ago until 1710.

They had scraped carvings of historic events, carvings that also described their spiritual faith. It was difficult for me to walk over the uneven steps on quartzite outcrops. A kind woman named Mary saw me struggle over the uneven rocks, and lent me her arm to keep from falling. Her kindness was much appreciated.

On our way to our night stay, we stopped at a place where a man by the name of Stan McCone had built a sod house similar to those built by some early homesteaders in 1880. It was on level ground, and quite solidly built; not much different from the root houses in Canada where they build small underground places to keep vegetables from freezing. They dug the ground four feet deep and two feet above ground level. It was covered with tree branches, straw and topped with soil. They were built in western Canada to keep potatoes and carrots from freezing in wintertime, at places where electricity was not available.

That evening we arrived at the Holiday Inn in the town called New ULM, in Minnesota. We stayed there for two days; the hotel was very comfortable with spacious rooms and beds.

Dinner was on our own which allowed us to get a meal of our choice. Sharing a table with two other sojourners, we enjoyed a class of wine with our dinner.

Wednesday June 9th Day three, on our vacation

Information about German Culture and Indian Wars:

In the morning we enjoyed a buffet breakfast, in the Mosel Danube Room in our hotel. There was a lot to eat, but my stomach was telling me to go easy on food because my stomach was not familiar with the different or somewhat strange German food.

Our first stop was visiting the "Brown County Museum" of German history in Minnesota: Germany was their former Fatherland.

The museum showed us from whence they came and their heritage with so many memories.

I was familiar with many of those articles as an immigrant myself from Holland: neighbor of Germany. I immigrated to Canada in 1948.

When I was looking around the museum, something was brewing in my mind. Memories prodded up about the Second World War when German soldiers occupied Holland. Then, when someone in this museum was going to give me a small sticker to put on my chest, it bothered me. I left the room to go outside. There was something that disturbed me, my memory in the past, when the Jews had to wear armbands with the name "Jew" to separate them from us whom they considered other (Germanic) Dutch people.

The next stop we visited was a newly built college chapel at Martin Luther College. While traveling towards the church on our bus we had a professor from the Martin Luther College who taught history of the German immigration and the background and inhabitants in Minnesota and the town of New ULM. He was very knowledgeable and could not stop telling his stories about German history and Indian wars. He spoke while the bus drove around to our next stop. I fretted but could not get out of the bus; he was driving me up a wall. I was stuck in the back of the bus and could not escape him. When we arrived at this most beautiful Lutheran chapel I made sure to stay in the back on a church bench so I could escape the professor's diatribe attack on my senses.

I fretted about myself: why I do not have more patience. Finally he stopped talking. Then the college organist played this beautiful very large pipe organ with songs so wonderful. Peace came in my heart and I thanked God for his patience with me, being a "Restless Traveler." Those familiar songs released my anxiety

Henceforth we were transported to the Shell Brewery: founded in 1866 by German immigrants. The name brewery sounded very interesting.

After being let through the factory and its more than a hundred year history, we were invited to their Tap Room.

We were invited to taste small amounts of different types of beer. It tasted good and put me in a mood to sing a song from my younger days. Not quite beholden for elderly Christian persons perhaps, but seemed funny.

Wednesday Eve

After a wonderful dinner at the Mosel Danube Room, still in New ULM, we were entertained by the "Concord Singers:" memorable German entertainment. I had hoped to read a few of my stories from my book called "Journal of a Dutch Immigrant" but there was no opportunity, so I sulked for a while until the twenty German Concord Singers started their program. Once they started singing, it reminded me of the time I was in Germany with my brother when we attended a similar musical entertainment, a place where every one was invited to join the singers. This time, too, I sang along. The music softened my disappointment of not a having a change to tell my story. The music moved me to the next bit of entertainment. A dozen characters, men and women, although difficult to distinguish because they were wearing wooden masks and colorful costumes. They entered the hall dancing and hobbled in between our dinner tables, encouraging us to join them. It took me a while before I was ready to accept their invitation: until I secured a woman who was a good dancer. I managed to get a hold of her. Her mask was not as scary as other ones. When the music stopped, she gave me a complement about my dancing. It made my day. That finished the evening; I enjoyed the camaraderie with our team of joyful vacationers, sharing our Christian fellowship with a delightful group of wonderful people.

Thursday June 10

Story telling by Jim Schaap about the 1862 Massacre, in Lower Sioux and South Dakota:

Jim has a knack in story telling that made us listen and hold our breath.

He had made an intense study of the wars between the Native Americans, also known as Indians, especially how white people from foreign countries gradually took over land that used to be Indian Territory, where they hunted buffalo, and were able to fish, and eat from other natural food that grew in that area. The white man, farmers, gradually built fences around their homesteads crowding the Natives away from their former land. Although many Natives were kind and even accepted the Christian faith, others became hostile and forced the others to join them in war against the settlers.

Jim came to the conclusion that eventually neither side was considered the winner in this war. So the Christian median could not say: who is to blame for this terrible end of bloodshed on both sides.

Friday June 11.

I was awakened by the telephone from the front desk at the Buffalo Ridge Resort called "Herrick Hotel" in Gary, South Dakota which was once a home for the blind and visually impaired. There were three buildings connected by underground tunnels for the blind students to move from the dorm to the dining room or class. It was closed some years ago, but bought by an investor who restored it into a business centre named Buffalo Ridge Resort. A delightful place to stay for a summer outing or to enjoy the campground next-door or go for a swim or boating.

9.15 Am. Off we went, going south to Palisades State Park: a unique area in South Dakota. There we saw the Sioux quartzite formation of Split Rock. The park is known for being where, once, "Jesse James" made his infamous "Out-law leap."

James Schaap delivered some exiting stories on Blue Mound Park where his close friend, "Frederick Manfred," author of several books, once lived. He built a house on the heights of the park so he could see the beautiful scenery below him.

From there we drove to Luverne in Minnesota. There we were invited to see the buffalo roam on a private ranch.

We were transported out to the buffalo herd on a hayrack with bales of straw to sit on or stand on a flat part of the hayrack. It was pulled by a tractor driven by the father of our host who was 97 years old, but doing fine.

I was not quite comfortable when we reached the herd of buffalo since my experience in our buffalo park near our city in the province of Alberta was different. There buffalo roamed freely and could attack you when getting close to them. I know of a friend who was attacked and was hospitalized for several days. However at this ranch the buffalo were used to visitors sitting on hayracks visiting them. We could reach out to them, handing them small rolls of crunched corn food.

After a lunch, consisting of buffalo meat on a bun, we left and headed for Worthington, Minnesota's Christian Reformed Church where we were entertained by six types of dishes cooked by people from different foreign backgrounds: a few from Sudan and China as well as others who made a dish of their choice; food from the country where they were born. They shared their native cooking skills. Most of them worked in a factory nearby and were invited to the church in Worthington which has been a blessing for them and the congregation.

It was time to head home: first to Dordt College for our go-away meetings where everyone could make comments or share their feelings about the trip.

For me it was a blessing to be together with persons I never met before because they were Christians who grew up in the faith as I was. I felt to be one, as brothers and sisters, with all who enjoyed this spectacular outing.

"The Restless Traveler"

By Jim Schaap

Somehow, I think I knew what was going on, in part, I think, because I knew the man, his history, and the sometimes stinging effects of childhood experience. He'd immigrated to Canada after the war, after the Nazi occupation of the Netherlands, and not all of that experience--hiding from conscription, living in fear day and night, the hunger winter--not all of that simply sifts out of one's life when it's left behind. If there are jackboots on the necks of your neighbors, you don't walk away whistling.

What happened was a kindly old retired professor walked up on the steps of the tour bus and began to tell the peculiarly German story of New Ulm, Minnesota, a town that celebrates its heritage of sauerbraten, schweinhocks, and polka bands. In his defense, the old prof was German-American, not German. In all likelihood, he spent the early 40s here in the States, picking ripened milkweed pods for parachute silk in the U. S. war effort, no more a Nazi than any of the other seniors on the tour bus.

No matter. Once he started talking--even though he spoke English with no accent--he was unapologetically German; after all, his chamber-of-commerce job was to sell the town, which means to sell the local, proud German heritage.

And our tourist, the man who couldn't forget the Nazis snarls in his boyhood backyard, got what the Dutch might call "benawed," so breathtakingly claustrophobic that he literally couldn't stand it. This 80+ year old war survivor had distinguished himself already as someone who could be strong-willed, to say the least. He was, after all, a man who'd climbed the Himalayas--no marshmellow. And he'd lost a leg in an accident--he hobbled demonstrably, but never complained. In just two days, he'd distinguished himself clearly, so when we noticed that something was decidedly wrong with him, initially at least, we rolled our eyes.

But my suspicions weren't far afield. Here's what he wrote in a little summary he penned of his experience on our Minnesota bus tour: "Memories podded up about the Second World War, when German soldiers occupied Holland--us. Then when someone was going to give me a small sticker to put on my chest, it bothered me. I left the room to go outside. There was something that disturbed me, my memory in the past, when the Jews had to wear are armbands with the name "Jew", to separate them from (us) whom they considered other (Germanic) Dutch people."

I think it was a version of post-survival stress. Something in the kindly old professor's mannerisms, his tone, his story, something in that little tourist sticker unearthed memories our own "restless traveler" might well have thought buried, and he nearly fell apart.

"He was very knowledgeable and could not stop telling his stories about German history and Indian wars," he wrote. "He spoke while the bus drove around, to our next stop. I fretted, but I could not get out of the bus; He was driving me up the wall. I was stuck in the back of the bus and could not escape him."

Achingly, painfully tethered. By choice, right then, he would have deserted the whole bus if he could avoid pain that was closing in on him--ancient, deadly fears long ago thought put to rest, but suddenly awakened by tone and rhetoric and ethnic pride.

When we got out of the bus at the new college chapel, I could see he was not to be reasoned with. Some spirit in him was out of control--and he knew it too. "When we arrived at this most beautiful Lutheran chapel," he wrote, "I made sure to stay in the back on a church bench, so I could escape the professor's diatribe attack on my senses. I fretted about myself--within my own, why I do not have more patience."

And then, "Finally he stopped talking," the Dutchman wrote.

The retired prof had stopped because we'd entered the Martin Luther College chapel, where, serendipitously, which is to say, providentially, the college's own fine organist just happened to show up. That man opened up that new huge organ in a fashion that no guitar and drum set can ever do. Together, we sang old hymns, even "A Mighty Fortress," Luther's own. It was a blessing I cannot describe. But our war survivor tries-- listen:

"Then the college organist played this beautiful very large pipe organ, with songs so wonderful. Peace came in my heart, and I thanked God for his patience with me, being a 'Restless Traveler.' Those familiar songs, released my anxiety," he wrote.

Those old hymns faith were decidedly providential therapy.

What he required at that point--and he understood it himself--was therapy. That retired history prof never wore the black SS coat and had nothing to do with The Final Solution.

He was an American, doing what lots of us do--taking pride in his heritage, including the town's own history, which started a full century before a little madman with a paintbrush mustache.

But there's a little more to the story of our restless traveler. Henceforth we were transported to the Shell Brewery, where, following a short tour, we were led thirstily to their tasting room for some product research.

"We were invited to taste small amounts of different types of beer," our restless traveler wrote, quelling, for a moment at least, his old fears and hatred. "It tasted good and put me in a mood to sing a song, song from my younger days--not quite proper for elderly Christian persons perhaps, but seemed funny." There's nothing like a little sip to help you forget, maybe, eh?

But the charmer was the evening, when, accompanying some fine German drinking songs, a motley crew of masked intruders, the Naaren, ended our German dinner by pulling every last one of the weary travelers from their chairs and waltzing them into a series of hoopla dances and marches that would have sent all of our travelers reeling had they carted in a keg or two with them. Which they hadn't, thank goodness.

Here's the way the Dutchman described the hijinks: "A dozen characters, men and women, although whether man and woman was difficult to distinguish, were wearing wooden masks and colorful costumes. They entered the hall dancing, and hobbled between our dinner tables, encouraging us to join. It took me a while before I was ready to accept their invitation, until I secured a woman who was a good dancer. I managed to get a hold of her. Her mask was not as scary as than other ones. When the music stopped, she gave me complement about my dancing. It made my day."

It made his day.

And thus, presumably, our restless traveler, so struck earlier in the day, was comforted finally, by the great hymns of the church, a few sips of good stout German beer, and a sporty jaunt with a masked intruder--a woman he managed to get hold of, he says, who then told him that for an old guy with a wooden leg, he was, by cracky, one heckuva good dancer.

And that's the whole story. Let preachers of all types and persuasions do with it what they will. All I know is, that's the way I saw it, and the way he tells it. There's got to be a sermon there, if we have ears.

Creation Awareness and Camping

Friday 4.30 PM: Just put up my tent between some trees on the property of a Bed and Breakfast place on a lonely stretch of road south of Bragg Creek or about 100 KM south west of Calgary. All campgrounds around the area are full due to a long weekend coming up. The mosquitoes are in full force and hungry for my blood. I seem to taste good because I can't keep them away. I will need some mosquito spray to prevent myself from going crazy.

My wife Grace and I traveled to Calgary the day before and stayed there overnight with Sherry de Roos. Grace wanted to shop with her sister Sherry for a day and I decided to revisit some beautiful country where, besides ranches and farms, also bear and cougar have their habitat.

Since I had become an amputee in 1987 I had dreams of camping and decided to go camping in the foothills of Alberta which is incredibly beautiful.

I traveled from Calgary west on Highway #8 the south on #22 to Bragg Creek, thence west on #66 to Elbow Falls enjoying the scenery of forested hills with many campgrounds which I investigated for a possible overnight stay. Since it was still before noon, I thought to return later to make suitable choice. I wanted to visit the "Bar U" Ranch first, some 60 KM further south.

This whole route going south on # 22 and side roads going west you witness these beautiful green pastures and forested hills as far as the eye can see and beyond that you see the majestic snow-capped Kananaskis Mountains.

The highlight was to view the Historical Bar U Ranch that was started in 1880 by a rich family from eastern Canada who had leased this land from the Canadian government: 157000 acres (or 63000 hectares). This place is just south of Longview. In 1890 they had over 10000 head of cattle and over 800 horses on their property. The cattle were raised for meat and the horses for racing and workhorses. Later this ranch was divided into 6 smaller ranches and in 1991 a small parcel of 140 hectares became a historical place of interest where you can still view the old ranch house and other buildings.

You can get a guided tour riding on a historical hayrack pulled by a pair of gleaming black horses. The smell of leather, on the harnesses, revisited my senses to an earlier time when I first came to Canada in 1948. I worked with an identical hayrack and horses for my uncle on a small ranch in mixed farming of grains and hay as well as cattle that roamed free in the daytime on open ranch land. In the evening after supper, I had to herd them back to the home corral. I rode a special trained horse called Peter (maybe he was named after my uncle who has that name). If a cow wandered off on its own and you steered the horse in its direction he knew what to do: this horse would race after it and get him back on track with the rest of the cattle. He was a joy to ride; I often rode him bareback like the Indians used to.

It is now 6.30m PM and I finished my supper consisting of a marinated rib-eye steak. My host at the Bed and Breakfast place invited me to use his gas fired barbecue in his back yard to cook my steak since there was no fire pit to cook as you normally have in campgrounds. I cooked it medium rare and instead of vegetables I ate some rye bread with it and a can of Beer to help it down the throat with a banana for dessert: most delicious.

Why was I camping in a tent by myself you might ask? Nostalgia!

40 years ago we used to go tent camping with our children; some years later it was a tent trailer, followed by a complete trailer with a bathroom and running water when our children got older and since Grace was not in love with mosquitoes: these pesky bugs that used to and still love her blood. Neither did Grace like the idea of meeting bears so I took up backpacking and once took our two oldest daughters along on some mountain trails which we enjoyed very much. Later on, when all had their jobs and got married, I went by myself and enjoyed meeting other hikers on my trails, sharing experiences. All that hiking ended when I became an amputee due to a cycling accident. Since then my camping gear had been in storage; gradually parting with most of the equipment over time but keeping my favorite little pup-tent and a sleeping bag that I used for some 20 years. Now and then I looked at it wondering whether I would ever use it again. I finally made the decision to go for it and here I am, taking my tent along on this expedition. My last Hurrah you might say, after which I will give away these last camping articles.

To my friends who asked the question: why are you going camping by yourself, such a lonely undertaking, my answer was: "I intend to Meditate." I thought it would be good to be alone and think about my past and have some spiritual meditation in the process. They thought I intended to read the Bible and pray all day, but that was not what I had in mind. It was more my wanting to re-experience the glory of God's creation, viewing his handiwork in the foothills of Alberta with the mountains in the background. It has such splendid vistas you cannot help but praise God for the wonders he created.

Then there is the matter of aging, I suppose it is like menopause: you don't have the vigor and energy anymore. There is still so much to do, see and experience. I noticed that with my friend Peter (5 years my senior) with whom I traveled through China and Middle Asia. He too had so many plans yet to realize: plans that had been on hold while he looked after his handicapped spouse before she went to Heaven.

Suddenly you find yourself slowing down, like the spirit is willing but your body says; please slow down. Getting slower on foot, having slower reactions and shorter memories; physical problems too: hearing is impaired, eyesight diminishing and skin cancer shows up. What is next, I wonder.

Still I am very thankful for love of family and friends; for God our creator of our beautiful earth (incidentally we are not taking very good care of our earth).

I am thankful for Jesus who paid for the mistakes I made in my life; Christ who understands my weaknesses and says: "Stick with me Francis. Just believe in me. Confess your mistakes and I will make you whole, like a spring chicken, but you have to wait a while. I am not ready to come down to earth yet."

Saturday morning June 29

I survived the night in my tent after 4 hours of sleep. I bedded down around 10.30 in the evening. Soon after undressing and getting comfortable in my sleeping bag, the zipper did not work. I tried to fix it, holding a small flashlight between my teeth but to no avail. I gave up and tried to go to sleep.

I thought if I could just fold the sack around me, it might work. No Sir! When you wish to turn around, part of your body becomes exposed and you get cold.

Fortunately I had a spare sleeping bag in the trunk of my car. I hated the idea of getting out of my tent, having to put my prosthetic leg back on, then get some clothes on... there was no other way out. In the meantime, an hour had passed and it was getting near midnight. After getting my other sleeping bag into the tent and getting comfortable inside it, my bladder told me to void some beer that I had consumed earlier. Fact is my Bed & Breakfast host offered me a beer while sitting around the fire pit. It always takes some time for it to filter through your kidneys and now it was time.

What horror: I had to get up again and drain the stuff out. It was probably after one o'clock that I finally dosed off until the morning light started to filter through the tent at 5.30. I opened my eyes, looked at my watch and thought: not yet, it is too early to get up. However, the birds started singing their morning song and I knew by 6 am I might as well break camp.

I arrived back in Calgary around 8.30 after stopping for breakfast in Bragg Creek. I picked up Grace who had enjoyed her shopping trip with her sister--telling proof: she carried a number of parcels into the car. We drove home with happy hearts.

Renaissance in Italy

A little background information: When the Kings University College opened its doors in September 1979 I decided to be one of its first students. In preparation for this exciting venture, I bought a book that related to my interest in European history and started to read. This got me so excited, I decided to visit Europe. Before classes started in September I took a Euro train tour to parts of Europe.

I spent most of my time in Florence, Italy where I boarded in a back alley home and shared a bedroom with two younger people, one from England and the other one from Germany. To get acquainted with the city, I headed for the palace of Lorenzo the Magnificent (Medici) of the 15th century. Lorenzo was very wealthy in his day and had become an unofficial ruler of Florence. Not being an appointed ruler, he was accepted as the best person with more experience as the ruler of the City of Florence.

Lorenzo was well educated, a free thinker who shared his thoughts. He was best known as a poet, connoisseur and lavish benefactor of art and learning. He was also a humanist, in contrast to his contemporaries, who lived under the rule of the Roman Catholic Church. This caused upheaval in Italy and prompted a priest called Savonarola to become his enemy. Many Florentines were troubled by the worldliness and paganism of the 15th century. I was captivated by Lorenzo, in the way he treated his fellowman, especially his generosity towards artists whom he invited to his palace where they could paint their pictures in his back yard garden. He had consideration for the underdogs: those who lived with little income.

The following day I went to visit the church where Lorenzo faithfully attended.

It surprised me that Lorenzo would attend the church where Savonarola preached, whose ideology was in stark contrast to Lorenzo's ideas of freedom of expression. Looking around the church, I met a guide who told me where Lorenzo usually sat and where he was attacked with a knife by a jealous business man. Lorenzo was protected from harm by his body guard. I wondered about the ideological struggle and the difficulty of the people in getting away from the power of the church.

His pastor got involved in politics. Savonarola was a great orator who criticized the humanistic direction which eventually caused Lorenzo to be discharged by the citizens of Florence who asked Savonarola to take over the duties of the head of Florence. However, his political involvement was not helpful. He had no experience in ruling the city. So the people of Florence burned him on a stake in 1498.

In the meantime, outside Italy, the renaissance continued in Western Europe. Erasmus of Rotterdam became the spokesperson of the intellectuals. He regarded the Middle Ages as a time of intellectual darkness and ridiculed the scholastic philosophers. Erasmus was keenly aware of the need to reform the clergy. He realized that the clergy and business are two different responsibilities. Erasmus put his faith in education and in enlightened discussion. He was against all violence or fanatics. He was urged to re-write the New Testament in the vernacular languages for better understanding of Christ's teachings.

From there on in it was Martin Luther, a monk, who had an introspective personality. He suffered from a chronic conviction that he was damned. By reading Romans 1:17, Martin Luther read "The just shall live by faith" which gave him relief. "Man could not earn salvation."

Then Calvin went a step further. Calvin agreed with Luther that justification is by faith and not by works. But they had a difference of opinion about predestination.

Both Calvin and Luther drew heavily on St. Augustine (420 ad) and his position on what God is expecting from his children. He too had a philosophy of dualism, drawing a split between what was earthly and what was from another world, one that was enduring, that is, a heavenly home.

By this time, I was at a loss, there seems to be no coming together in faith. There was more competition between churches than working together for the better way of expressing God's promises for his people. After this trip, I returned home somewhat depressed, but felt consoled in that there is a time to come when we will be rejoicing in a perfect world with no ending.

Part Two: Poetry

Catching up at Fifty

Sabbatical
Hungering
For knowledge
Kings Universiy

Money by itself
No satisfaction
Seeking enrichment
University college

Was welcomed
By youngsters
Half my age
Showing Interest
In this Elder
With respect

Fellow Sojourners
New endeavors
What's to come?
Setting goals

Eagerness
Get acquainted
With the world
And its past

Seeking directions
Where have we been?
Where are we going?
In years to come

Spirit of adventure
Studying History
About the world
And it's struggles
Writing Essays
Philosophy
Languages
Theology

Endless studies
About
Ancient times
Roman Empire
Greece, Rome
Christianity

Middle Age
Florence Italy
Power Struggles
Papal rule

Savonarola *
Versus
Lorenzo *
Poet and Ruler

Renaissance
Upheaval
Separation
Church and state

Erasmus *
Explanations
Luther &Calvin
Different insights

No peace on earth
War and destruction
Lord help us
We need you.

*Savonarola—1498 Priest
*Lorenzo 1449–1492
*Erasmus 1497–1543

Aging

A three quarter century
That is me Today
The twenty fourth of May

Seventy-five years went by
And here am I
Leaving so much behind
Hope the future will be kind

In nineteen twenty nine
First saw light to shine
Upon this world in its time,
Not everything quite divine

In retrospect I had great respect
Parents demonstrating what's correct
Showing direction towards a destination
Of learning the truth by observation

Attending a Christian school that could
Teach you what is wrong, what is good
To discern the truth and therein
Maturing in wisdom and discipline

Back to aging, getting old
Until now I felt quite bold
Not ready to slow down
Often playing the clown

Athletic I was, going gung Ho
Loving outdoor activities and so
Running, Hiking and cycling
Until hit by a car while biking *

As a result became an amputee
Lost my leg below the knee
Being an optimist I had trust
To overcome obstacles or bust

Grace had petitioned heavens gate
My husband is too fast, I am afraid
Please give him some direction
Before I loose him and his affection

His answer gave her a fright
But I assured her she was right
The accident I underwent
Was not necessarily Gods intent

Together we faced the world anew
I used crutches and canes we flew
To Holland first then unto Arizona
Our winter home with its Bon Vista

All was well and seemed serene
We thought what does that mean
When over time two brothers died
Then a sister, it gave us fright

Frailty is staring us in the face
And we must be ready in case
Our Lord is calling us home
Meeting him before his throne

So when something goes wrong
Do not forget a praising song
Your pain, and losing eyesight too
God knows, he will take care of you

Maybe our future is not sure
But we do feel secure
God will hold us by his hand
Preparing us for his Fatherland

Apache Junction AZ

We love our home

While I sit on my throne
Inner self tells me to move
Where weather will improve
Before becoming discontent
Reason is irrelevant
Within me, there is an alarm
Go to where it is warm.

Once I feel this drive
I am feeling more alive
Move to Arizona, bite the dust
To satisfy your wanderlust

Apache Junction, is our sanctuary
Weather, milder there in January
Our favourite palm tree is there
A resting place in a rocking chair

Come spring there is the call of Geese
They are heading for the River peace
Sun is rising come with us please
Temperature there will increase

We felt, we were young
Insurance says; you are wrong
The gong will sound are long
Your life will not prolong.

Back Packing

The north boundary trail

Not for someone frail
A hundred mile distance without news
Wonderful trip with spectacular views

Trekking mile after mile
Resting so once in a while
Enjoying our food at even tide
See the Sun, watching its slide

Pitching up our cozy tent
Recording the days event
Once we turned very pale
Leaft no breath to inhale

A wolf was on our path
Showed no interest or wrath
We looked her in the eye
She blinked and went by

Continuing on our trail
While walking in the dale
Virgin forest so peaceful and still
Intercepted by birds their shrill

It was the grandest tour
Hiking on rough contour
Some trees are quite tall
Made us feel very small

Passing a lake to be sure
Made the choice to detour
Crossing a fast running creek
Fridgit, scary, made us weep

Mornings awakened without a clock
Squirrels came down to knock
Dropping pinecones on our tent
Birds sang to their hearts content

Crossing the Snake Indian Pass
Half waypoint, with ice likes glass
We're at our greatest height
Without mosquito that bite

The sky was heavenly blue
Then snow, not to look forward to
On that eve we made a roaring fire
Dried our clothes, strung on a wire

Once a porcupine sitting in the wood
Was biting my salted marianted boot
Wanted to kick him, if I could
His needles, doubted if I should

All part of God's creation
His wilds a demonstration
Inviting us to participate
Meditating on His real estate

Drinking in its beauty and all
With musical insects very small
Wild flowers that inbreed
Poppies not quite pedigreed

Day Ten, down hill in euphoria
To our car and off to Victoria *
First to restaurant for a big meal
Poor waitress, our smell had no appeal

*Edmonton 1974

Bangladesh

Roy and Grace
Did embrace
Finding space
In Bangladesh

Working days
By Gods Grace
Children to bless
In Bangladesh

They are Passionate
Teaching the illiterate
Literacy they confess
Needed in Bangladesh

Roy undertakes a deed
With urgency and speed
Fulfilling a special need
In Bangladesh

His helpmate Grace
Supporting him in ways
And Deserves much praise
In Bangladesh

To reach the poor
In Christ's name to score
Souls for heaven's door
In Bangladesh

Bicycle Dream '87

Blessed with a body healthy and strong

I loved exercise-it couldn't go wrong
Running did the trick until
The knees cried out "We're getting sick"

Heeding the body' lament
A Mountain bike kept me content
Keeping the body physically fit
Cycling became my sport, testing it

With effort, lost weight, felt hard-pressed
Racing fellow bikers, to stay abreast
Pedaling through the countryside
Enjoying the flowers at harvest time

Dreamed of cycling to the Pacific coast
Vancouver to be my winning post
Obtaining a bike to cycle and race
That long distance at a steady pace

It required time and a will to train
Cannot complain when cycling in rain
Must make a decision when to depart
Before I would lose heart

Cycled an eight hour day
Visiting a daughter, hundred miles away
Edmonton to Neerlandia, seemed so far
Pedaling to Vancouver better to take the car

Arriving sweaty and drained
My buttocks somewhat pained
My grandson questioned the episode
And said: But Grandpa you're old!

One monday my wife and I picked beans
And canned them, all is well it seems
I went for bike ride, had no doubt
To return, but got a wiped out

Police officer came to our door
Come to Hospital, there is more
Will call your children to be sure
Come and see if there is a cure

That accident took my dreams away
Had no recollection I could not say
Was informed the following day
Hit by someone, who did not make way

I awoke in the Hospital delirious
Wishing healing not to be serious
Pain and confusion were there
But I felt surrounded by prayer

It gave me peace, I ask not why
Church community, reached the sky
Body and mind were now at peace
Doctors, Nurses worked without cease

I was weakened, tearful from operations
Doctor Wilkes showed me his creation
With other body parts to annex
He rebuild the Leg restored the reflex

Covered the wound, grafted the skin
From the other leg, very thin
Over time sufficiently recovered
Thanked God and prayers offered

Once removed from this sting
I was sure the future would bring
Relief I would be going full swing
Surprised, now moving on a wing

PS: Became a below knee amputee

Boasting

I was the man who used to boast
That I could do the uttermost
Someday! But I did not know
How to keep my brain in tow

Therefore a laborer now I am
Nothing came forth of an earlier plan
To become rich and well to do
Now am the keeper of an animal zoo

Christmas 2009

Jesus is born
Who is he then?
Son of God
To do what?
Save his people
From whom?
The Evil one

You know him?
Yes he is mean
In which way?
Destroying us
How?

Long story
Was an Angel
Became jealous
Hates God
Wants to Destroy
This beautiful world
And mislead
God's Children
That is Us
Using subterfuge
Making us believe
Its Ok to:

Being selfish
Envying your neighbour
Steal their possessions
Misusing power
And much more
How do you know?

I Read the Bible
Our world was perfect
It belongs to God
He wants to rescue us
From the evil one
By sending Jesus
Who loves us
He gave his life

For us to live
In a world to come
Called Heaven
A peaceful place
Indescribable
Beautiful
Jesus invites us
To his heaven
For those who
Follow his precept
Love your neighbour
As yourself

Ask Gods presence
In your life
Join us
It's Christ's Birthday
Two thousand years
A multitude of Angles
In the sky
Welcomed Christ
Presently In Heaven
Where God reigns

There will come a day
The Prince of peace
Will come back
To this Earth
To rescue us
From the one
Causing destruction
Of God's World
Amen

Creation Awareness

The earth was created by God
Where man and woman may trod
Where do we get this information?
The Bible reveals this creation.

God created mountains and flatlands
With Maples, viola's, and other plants
Fish in the waters and birds in the air
And a host of different animals in pairs.

With harmony between man and beast
Adam was the first-born, God's priest
He gave names to animals and birds
Rain was provided to quench thirst.

The earth was beautiful and serene
God then created Eve as Adam's queen
Later a fallen angel broke the spell
And God explained there would be Hell.

Division occurred between God and man
God did not come to visit, as was His plan
Did God arrange for earth's orbit to change?
Cause it to tilt, animals become deranged?

Despite changes in seasons and weather
From unknown climates before, we gather
The earth still provided food and water
And man could use animals for slaughter.

Human species survived and tilled the earth
With sweat on their brow, as man was cursed
For centuries there was an ecological balance
Though keeping it good was a big challenge.

God gave man intellect to gain
Knowledge to experiment and train
Animals for transport and heavy pulling
So mankind had more time for schooling.

In time man gained more intellect
Developed mechanisms having an effect
Caused a revolution, things mass produced
Products and gadgets for their ease in use.

Wealth and power now was pursued.
Me, Myself and I, became the attitude
Leisure, food and selfishness ensued
Resulting in a lack of gratitude

When twentieth century came around
Automobile developed caused a wound
Rich soil replaced with asphalt and tar
Leaving the earth with big ugly scars.

Large cities are built near water
And farmers are forced to scatter
Soil is replaced with highways to transport
Suburban dwellers to their city in comfort.

Now we have highways and byways
Cluttered with autos, trucks and strays
Spouting out toxins to foul the air
Resulting in people who die in despair.

We are despoiling the earth
Babes in the womb die before birth
We are becoming deaf and insane
"The the earth is groaning with pain."

Our quest for oil has made us blind
New resources we may not find
The need for more will create a war
Man may die for fuel in his car.

God is the creator, provider of all
Food for his creatures, great or small
He takes much pleasure when we care
For our fellow man, our willingness to share.

Lord have mercy on us in success
Our wealth gives us so much stress
We must seek your path and regain
An earth renewed, and a clean terrain.

* (Romans 8-22)

King's University College

My favorite subject was History
Not dwelling on people's misery
Rather it was about series of events
Of nations bent on destroying
Or conquering their fellow men
Most often in the name of God
I learned how utterly depraved we are
When craving Power and Gold
The study of History made me pause
How utterly dependent on God we are
The need to petition our Lord and King
To guide our lives in everything
Thank you professors you were

So gracious allowing me to earn
A Bachelor's degree in History
Thank God for the King's University College
From where I graduated I thought with polish

King's University College—Alternate Version

Subject is History
Serious events
Conquering
Each Other

People's misery
In gods name
Destroying
Themselves

Much depravity
Craving Power
And gold
Gave me pause

Utterly dependent
On god's grace
To be rescued
From ourselves

Professor in candid
Guiding us
Opening eyes
To be ready
It's your future

Dear Professor of Philosophy

For me Philosophy is treason
There is no rhyme or reason
Tangled language no conclusion
Just words flooding in profusion

Enclosed Socratic number Six
Slowly but surely I am getting a fix
On this difficult exercise
It's not my type of enterprise

Distraction becomes a big factor
My logic definitely a protractor
Cobwebs in my brain are thick
And you so eloquent and quick

With Russell, Moore and Lock
My thoughts are on the clock
In philosophy I'm not a bloomer
Thank you for your good humor

You taught me in good cheer
I'll accept you as my peer

Cuban experience 1998

Always had the urge
So I could emerge
And be informed
Christians there Reformed

booked a flight
And so I might
Visit the Isle of Cuba
Ninety miles from Florida

Cuban's resources, sugar and fruit
With tourist dollars to boot
Governed by a regime malign
Other say Castro is benign

Under one party rule
Indoctrinated in school
In Marxist ideology
No tolerance for diversity

Tourist flock to island beaches
No interest in Cuba's (human) creatures
What their plight might be
Or to go with them on bending knee

Tourist, eat, drink and devour
Dollars keeps Castro in power
Its habitants are resigned
To the facts of live and grind

Yet greet you with a smile
While visiting their Isle
My brother and I enjoyed our stay
Were privileged to visit and pray
With friends seeking a destiny
Sharing the gospel in their society

The Cubans love music and song
You cannot help but join the throng
It was so in my situation
Towards the end of my vacation

I had a dance with music sublime
A Chambermaid, bodies in rhyme
Thanked her having danced with me
With this old man, an amputee.

Elton John

On a cruise ship
Entertained us
On a Piano
Wearing sunglasses

Wearing a white jacket
Baring his Chest
Wearing high heels
Bouncing the Piano
Bellowing a song
And is clowning

This is our
Young Generation
Likes to scream

Aging Attendees
Shaking their heads
About the new age
And its artistic art
Of the day

Friday 1987

Cycling
The Dreamer
Edmonton
Vancouver
700 Miles

Weekend
Testing
Strength
Distance

Sun rise
Two Hours
Breakfast
25 miles

Short sleeves
Elevation
Creek
Fifty

Ten thirty am
Red scarf
On the level
Surrounded

Potato fields
Rolls of hay
Yellow fields
Seventy five

Take a break
Ham and cheese
Making time
Neerlandia
One Hundred

Monday Following

Sunny day
The garden
Green Beans
Kitchen
Canning

Eleven Am
Back in an hour
Usual route
Knock on door

Officer
Missericordia
Loved ones
Come as you are
Your Pastor too

Automobile
Bicycle
Catapult
In ditch

Eventide
Family together
Many wires
Morphine
Why?

Surgery
Eight hours
Six weeks
No success

Twice repeated
Sixteen month
Decision made
Left below
Amputee

Grace's 80ᵗʰ Birthday

Happy Birthday Grace
With your smiling face
For 80 years you're on the go
And your face is still aglow
You walk a fifteen-minute mile
Greeting every one with a smile
Leaves her husband way behind
With his cane, walking is a grind
She cooks his dinners, so divine
While we share a glass of wine
Husband prefers a New York steak
With mushrooms, he's wide-awake
She keeps her husband on the roll
In a subtle ways she keeps control
Grace your attributes are many
Especially in the role of granny
To her grand children she is drawn
But needs to rest when they are gone.
By Gods Grace we are together yet
With my impatience, I feel in debt
Love you dear, let us cheer
Happy Birthday Grace my dear

*September 8, 2007

Handicapped

I am an amputee
Left below the knee
Not quite obvious to see
Trousers cover the injury
It takes an expert eye
Must be observant like a spy

I am content despite my situation
Experiencing days of some frustration
Climbed the Acropolis to its height
In Greece, without too much fright
Reaching the Parthenon and stood
On rocky ground, and felt hard put

Walking is becoming a bit slow
In earlier days I ran like a doe
Long distance running, I ran with ease
Ligaments cried out, especially the knees
I didn't know what it was like to go slow
Stopped in my tracks some years ago
Backpacking was my favorite sport
It required strong legs to support
A pack of food, sleeping bag and tent
Some paraphernalia within its content

One summer, I canoed to the Arctic coast
A long story, I don't want to boast
From Lac de Grass to Coppermine
Paddled 400 miles in four weeks time

Disability can have its compensation too
Once, traveled by wheelchair through
Four countries in coach, with first class care
Attendants pushed wheelchair without fanfare
Once was moved to a business class seat
To be close to toilet, stewards were so sweet

I was on crutches, people opened doors
Attentive to see if they could do more
Smiling, I said thank you, enjoyed the attention
My condition was obvious no need for pretension

It happened in 1987 while riding my bike
Hit from behind I became an airborne kite
Landed all bloody with the leg all torn
On a beautiful sunny day in the early morn
Not being conscious throughout the fray
Or expected to live out that day

Saved by the Grace of God, who lifted the curse
Of death; By an Angel in the form of a Nurse
Who saw it happening and stopped the bleeding

Transported to Hospital;
Ambulance Speeding

I was able to praise God for his care
Even though I was not yet aware
No more athletics except for swimming
A blessing in disguise, now always winning
Once entered the Arizona Senior Olympic
To swim a Mile in my age class to win *

Therefore I am grateful for stamina and will
And to this date am a regular swimmer still
No competition, with no one else in the Pool
To dream or pray for the day and feeling cool

*January 25, 2005
*1996-1500 meters, 31 minutes

Winter 1990

Healing
I declare do not despair
Surgeon: I will repair
No thoughts of defeat
Healing would be complete

Doctor sets bones
Strong like stones
Leg to mend
Might even bend

Doctor a technician
God the Physician
Doctors have talent
God has the patent

Creator and created
Not to be separated
We need them both
For healing and growth

To the therapist I go
Crutches through snow
Exercising with springs
And other implements

Therapist berates
Patient wants debate
How to proceed
With treatments

With aid of two canes
Thankfully mild pain
Moving at a slower pace
Without the briefcase

For additional therapy
I would travel to Hawaii
Sun and vitamin "D"
Swimming the deep blue sea

Optimism was premature
After the operation
I became a below knee amputee
There would be no Hawaii,
Or swimming in the deep blue sea

If At First You Don't Succeed—Try, Try Again

The theme for today is writing,
A project somewhat frightening,
Wanting to write a parable or a story
For acceptance, if not for glory.

Sometimes you might feel down or bent,
But never should you say, "I can't"
To writing that story or that Poem,
Feeling heavy hearted like a stone.

Away with thoughts of accepting defeat.
Keep on writing; you will succeed.
Then someone will say, "That is neat,"
Just the encouragement you need.

Just stop, give it some time, read a book—
Rest your mind; then take a second look.
Go away somewhere and dream away,
Meeting other people, who might say---

"I like it." With a positive attitude,
The mind becomes at ease, and feels good.
Therefore, you try again; do not despair.
New thoughts will come floating through the air.

Continue your journey with writing;
Never mind critique that's biting;
Write what's in your heart, words will flow like rain.
Try, try again; nothing comes without pain.

In the Deep

Releasing anxiety
Two arms, one leg
Arms plowing
Through the water
Lost time of day
Dreams of a future
Past and present
Will I be led?

Future excitements
Challenging
Ride a balloon
Studying the Moon?
Write a Poem
A Haiku Tune?
Swim like a fool
Fulfilling a duel?

Where is he now
Did he shed a tear
Twenty years ago
Leaving one to die

Along the Road

In tall grass
Was there remorse?
In his dreams?

A Nurse
From a distance saw
Biker Catapulted
Left in the ditch
Aid administrated
Infirmary
Will he live?
Yes, I am here

Change in Life

It was me
In the limelight
It was I
Who had forthright?

It was me
Who drove the car
It was I
Who became marred

It is she
Who is in charge
And for Me
To go and march

It is I
Now watch the sky
No more me me and I

It is She
Who's defined
Who loves me
And is very kind

King's University College

Subject is History
Serious events
Conquering
Each Other

People's misery
In gods name
Destroying
Themselves

Much depravity
Craving Power
And gold
Gave me pause

Utterly dependent
On god's grace
To be rescued
From ourselves

Professor in candid
Guiding us
Opening eyes
To be ready
It's your future

I visited my nephew near La Rochelle, France
He has a small Estate called: La Tourtelle
Andre has no title, he represents a seed company.

La Tourtelle

La Maison de Marqui
A proper place you will agree
For Lord Andre` and his Queen
Who goes by the name Sabrine

Taken possession of this property
To provide a Home and stability
And a place to start a family
Where Ambre` made it a Trinity

With Les Chiens called Max and Molly
Together with three Cats the place is jolly
Chickens laying eggs for le Petite desjeuner
La Maison est complete ne outre pas desirer

The yard filled with flowers and trees
Makes it a sanctuary, a feeling of peace
Surrounded by a fence and a gate
With Dogs and Cats no reason to be afraid

Guests will be welcomed by Sabrine
And treated with a great cuisine
Lord Andre`will give you a tour
Few days later he'll say: Bon Jour

*June 2004

Lamentation

I Lament
I do not understand
Our World as it is
When seeking its bliss

I Lament
And do not understand
When Politicians doublespeak
Their message often reeks

I Lament
When the media portents
That they can make us wise
To the road to paradise

I Lament
When I cannot comprehend
Having no clue, what is true?
From what I hear or read
With information at high speed

I Lament
When encouraged to buy and spend
On articles: supposed to be God sent
Giving me unease, instead of peace

No more lament
Since God will make me content
He knows my needs better than I
So carry on, no need to cry
Thank you my Lord for being there
I speak to you; I know you care

Languages

The English language can be bothersome
When it is not your Mother tongue
English is my language of choice
Not many understand the other voice

I was born in the Netherlands
Dutch my first language you understand
In Holland I learned to twist my tongue
Into spoken words and jubilant song

In early age a restless student I was
Never an achiever in junior class
My innermost spirit running amok
Having so many playful visions in stock

Putting words into certain order
Was lost to me as so much bother
Since then I changed my attitude
Writing Poetry: to be understood

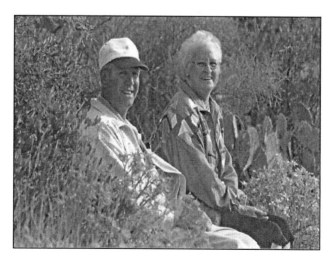

Latitude 34

Haven of Rest
Winter Home
Wearing shorts
Children Splashing
Colours everywhere
Poppies, Roses
Darkness to Light
Saturday night ball
Sunday Singing
Monday Tennis
Tuesday
Arts and Crafts
Full Moon
Coyote, Fox
Owls
Dawn
Bluebird and Blossoms
Morning Goldfinch
Carninal and Birch
Cactus in Bloom
Butterflies
Rattlesnakes
Sun and Shadow
Fulfilling

Luke 2

Once upon a time
2000 years ago
Emperor Augustus
The rural of Israel
Of the Jew's People
They were crying for help
And became very sorry, not
Having followed Gods advice
Then one day Shepherds
Where in the field
Watching the sky
Watching a thousands Angels
Praising God in Heavens
Saying, there will
be peace on earth.

Then the shepherds chanted
Hallelujah's many times.
Then the shepherds ran to
the town of Bethlehem
And found Mary and Joseph
With a child laying in a manger
Named Jesus

Then the shepherds returned to
the farm looking after their sheep
And were very happy and
kept Glorifying and praising
God for the promise
that there will be peace
On earth
Repeating the hallelujah's
Praising the master of the Universe

*Luke 2:1-20

Memoir at Eighty

From bold to old
Springbok to Turtle
Foxtrot to a Ballad
Decisive and Quick
While on my walk
Passed by a snail
Uses a Cane
Strong Opinion
I am not so sure
A large Home
Moved to Condo
Words we use
Beautiful and Sexy
Time goes by
Intelligent and Kind
Man's expectations
Age makes one wiser
I love you so dearly
So glad you are here
Let's celebrate
A hug and a kiss
Will be fine

My Dear Valentine

Grace you are
None holds Barr
Lover and friend
Keeping me content
Your' there for me
With coffee or Tea

I'm always on the go
There is no need to say no
I have lost my Libido
Our faces still glow

What else can I say?
We continue to play
Hide and seek
Shower and peek

We both look well
In clothes that tell
Beauty is in our sight
No change over night
Might grow older
But not boulder

My Memoir

Born in The Netherlands 1929
Small village, horticultural region
1940-45 Teenage years,
War, anxiety, curfews, fear

Grade six, teacher ex-sergeant, disciplinary
Grade eight, non-academic stream
Self-worth was impeded
Restless, loved play and games

1948 British Columbia, uncle, mixed farm,
Horses and cattle
Winter, bush, timber, sawmills

1952 Edmonton, my sister
Encouraged to read, learned new words
Canadian National Railway
Applied and declined, employment,
Apprenticed, no pay, was hired
Telegrapher, one year, laid off

1954 Applied sales position
Seed company five years, felt appreciated
1959 Recruited, sold Life Insurance
Discovery, I could absorb information
Did well, built vocabulary

1979 Money, by itself, no gratification
Applied to enter college, part time
Discovered my potential, sweating
Had the words, not right order, red ink

1987 Bachelor of Arts, in History
2003 Arizona College, read a Poem
Professor, much praise, shed a tear
2005 Here I am, Thank you Lord

My Sinful Life

It is about the mind within
Two spirits are dueling to win
The heart of human creatures
Made aware by preachers

The Bible tells the story
To find a heavenly glory
The opposite spirit is the snake
Will woo away, your God to forsake

The battle is a quest for souls
Each has difference goals
One for life to a heavenly realm
The other, death to overwhelm

Our creator made everything pure
For all his creatures to be secure
A fallen Angel put a rod in the spoke
But Christ made that angel to uncloak

Became aware of Heaven and Hell
The Angel of death has a dirty smell
Thrown out of heaven, forever to quell
Sent into the realm of darkness to dwell

Impatience might annoy
Someone you love and enjoy
Short temper could well impede
Longing for closeness to succeed

What is there to entice causing sin?
Hatred might just do a man in
Must exercise self- discipline
Murder, is not for the Born-again

If the above gives you a scare
Just be ready and then prepare
For Christ's return, confess your sin
He will have mercy and take you in

Patience

I never had any; and
If thoughts are worth a penny
Given time to think and reflect
Upon my past with due respect

Some years ago I had an accident
Since then I am more penitent
The Lord has given me much healing
If not the injury, then in my being

Thankful for the past,
Enjoying God's creation full blast
Canoed rivers, hiked mountains high,
Running and cycled under a blue sky.

I loved a challenge; true
Always looking for something new
But never thought I would be faced
With the challenge of constraint

Lord give me the courage once again
Since I have to endure much more pain
Please bless the prognosis by Dr.Savoy
My leg may heal and I its use enjoy

However it was not to be
I became a below knee, amputee
Comforting to know God shows the way
For me to be thankful every day

Dear Professor of Philosophy

For me Philosophy is treason
There is no rhyme or reason
Tangled language no conclusion
Just words flooding in profusion

Enclosed Socratic number Six
Slow but sure I am getting a fix
On this here difficult exercise
It's not my type of enterprise

Distraction becomes a big factor
My logic definitely a protractor
Cobwebs in my brain are thick
And you so eloquent and quick

With Russell, Moore and Lock
My thoughts are on the clock
In philosophy I'm not a bloomer
But thank you for good humor
Teaching me in good cheer
I'll accept you as my peer

Physical Therapy

Suffering from Osteo Arthritis
And things like Tendonitis
To a therapist I went
Arriving somewhat bent

Diagnosis completed they suggest
Lie down and get partly undressed
Was self conscious of my derrière
Gas might escape from my interior

What if therapist would faint?
Other patients had complained?
Fortunately I was able to contain
Explosive substances without pain

Therapist goes to work and smiles
Asks me to turn over; Her style
Take a deep breath; then exhale
Next you know your getting pale

Had difficulty to hold my tongue
For fear she'd pummel my bum
Specially this sensitive body part
Might produce a thunderous fart

Felt better after turns and twist
Thanks to Michelle my therapist
Being dismissed somewhat frail
Without leaving a vapour trail

Prayer for Reconciliation

Dear Heavenly Father and Lord
I read about your word
You the creator of the universe
Lifting us from the earthly curse

You will hold us if we pray
For salvation, your laws obey
Hear my prayer from a heavy heart
Please redeem me do not depart

I bare my soul and supplicate
The evil one might infiltrate
My soul and say, you are good
Come along get in the mood

Show the world how good you are
You don't steal, swear, or pilfer a car
Why not join us in the worldly bar
Have some fun, there is no war

Thank you Lord, you took control
With your spirit, you saved my soul.
Jesus died to pay for my sin
Baptized me for a new begin

I want to celebrate and raise
My voice to sing your praise
You have delivered me from guilt
Jesus, who's heavenly home is built

I rest secure, having faith in you*
Seeking Christ purpose for me and to
Continue daily life, no one can take away
Christ love and sanctification come what may.

Luke 5-20 NCRV
When he saw their faith, he said
"Friend, your sins are forgiven you"

Swimming

I went for a swim one day
In Edmonton's YMCA
Arizona I swam in an outdoor pool
Edmonton temperature is too cool
Prefer to swim in an early hour
When one has much more power
All lanes in the pool were in use
With joggers, not swimmers, obtuse
In one lane, I spied a lone swimmer
Looked like a mermaid but thinner
A woman graceful had a gentle stroke
Caused forgotten feelings to be evoked
"Beauty is in the eye of the beholder"
They say: As I who am getting older
Entranced I was, her grace and speed
Sliced the water: A Barracuda indeed
I entered the pool, goggles in place
Ready to swim and gave chase
Followed a creature well endowed
Goggles fogging up my snout
Did not prevent to dream away
Just allowed the image full sway
Thoughts encroaching in a way
Keeping sober preventing a fray
One needs an open mind I stress
Ambivelant thoughts make a mess
God's creation we should not miss
Allow ourselve its sights and bliss
Finished our swim with elation

Elicited a smile of appreciation
We'd swam in perfect formation
During a forty minutes duration

*May 2004

The Coppermine River Adventure

On the 12th of July 1982
From Yellowknife we flew
Due north to Lac de Grass
Canoeing a river raw

To our great surprise
The lake was full of ice
But upon closer scrutiny
In shore it was ice-free

We unloaded the twin Otter plane
To fly back to Yellowknife again
Left with only shrubbery to burn
A desolate place of no return

Five men and one woman strong
In three canoes, what could go wrong?
Only 400 miles paddling ahead
To Artic coast, no contact by Internet

Gordon, a teacher leading our troupe
Teachers: Robert and Les also in our group
Henry the Artist, Francis the wanderlust
Basia, a nurse and accomplished canoeist

Day one, dragging the canoe over ice
Then into clear water, that was nice
Setting up camp with mosquitoes unseen
Into our food, giving us free protein

Next day our first set of rapids to pass
With a wetsuit,mosquitoes stinging our ass
Canoes, dipping its nose into the waves
Scary at first, but we were braves

The headwaters of the Coppermine River
Were very cold, with bathing we shivered
The first week was sunny and warm
The countryside, though barren, had charm

Setting up camp at night was no big deal
The Wild Cat Café, was our last good meal
Still, we ate our meal with anticipation
Mosquito's sharing our meal without invitation

The vast Tundra had a spectacular view
With vegetation growing I never knew
Growing on permafrost one foot deep
Lunar landscape, beautiful, I could weep

Great expanse of rock and shrubs, no trees
Desolate, yet grandiose with undulated seas
With its organisms so pretty in all
Our creator at work, I felt so small

Many more rapids ahead to give us fright
Some dangerous, with no time for respite
We hated to portage it gave us pain
Carrying canoe and baggage seemed insane

Obstruction Rapids was a real challenge
Avoiding rocks, with waves to keep balance
The river zigzagged, it took much skill
To maneuver and paddle, and not to spill

With porridge in our belly, we brace
Big open lake waters and wind to face
Waves, got to a height, we took fright
Going helter-skelter but managed with pride

Next day it was sunny and bright
We paddled on Point Lake until night
Made good progress on this long lake
With enough time to cook and bake

One night we watched the midnight sun
Coming down over the water, there it clung
We tried to sleep in the open air
Mosquito's relentless, difficult to bare

ntering Coppermine River was a delight
The flow of water made paddling light
Until the rapids in a canyon did appear
Necessitating portage, and carry our gear

Ten days later our hearts skipped a beat
A floatplane went by looked real so neat
It landed a little down yonder
What could that be, we did wonder

Canoeist from the Minnesota state
Fresh and clean as if on a parade
We felt rugged, veterans very good
They were leaving for the river Hood

As a diversion from paddling and food
We fished to improve our diet and mood
Our supper made from a dehydrated dish
Was complemented with bannock and fish

We passed the Arctic Circle at 66 degrees
Most times we saw just low shrubs, no trees
Along the river shore we found wood galore
Making campsite fires easy on shore

An interlude along the river Coppermine
Maxwell Ward, entertained us, it was divine
It was his fishing tent camp, his hideaway
It kept his telephone and business at bay

Sometimes running high waves
We cried with delight willing to face
The waves to dip into while hit by spray
Like a bucking horse its rider made sway

Without serious incident to date
Entering Escape Rapids without debate
To check from shore, if there was threat
Not expecting this set of rapids as yet

Sometimes caution goes by the wind
Resulting in language not fit to print
Suddenly boulders and waves we faced
Rob & Les capsized, from drowning saved

We took a break, made fire to warm
The dunk-lings and all was calm
Ending the day with fish and caribou steak
A delicious meal that Basia did make

The end of our trip was coming near
We continued our voyage without fear
One obstacle, the Bloody Falls, was left
A dangerous set of rapids in a cleft

This place in 1772 where Samuel Hearne
Saw Dene Indians making Eskimos squirm
By killing them on a blood thirsty night
Giving Samuel Hearne his greatest fright

Reaching Coronation Gulf on Arctic coast
After four weeks of paddling we could boast
Survival on that arduous voyage by canoe
By the grace of God, this saying is true

Our tents on campground near our beach
Welcomed by Inuit and presented each
With the gift of some seal liver meat
Thankfully accepted, delicious, a treat

Our arrival at Coppermine town coincided
With Inuit Games and we were provided
Entertainment of Inuit culture and fare
Wonderful experience, glad we were there

Time to take flight we stayed overnight
At Yellowknife, the weather was bright
Morning church service about prodigal son

Thankful For Gods Grace,
That I Might Be One

Great to be home after 5 weeks absence
And what a joy to see family and friends
All was well, so many stories to tell
Now safe on deck, no shipwreck all is well

*August 2001

A Few Quotes from former Prime Minister Trudeau, Who Canoed This River in 1944

"Its such a pleasure when you draw a deep breath of rich morning air right through your body, after a cold night curled up like an unborn child."

"You return not so much as a man of reason, but a more reasonable man."

The Love of My Life

It was in nineteen fifty-five
When I met my darling wife,
Taking notice of her one day
Walking with her elegant sway
Transfixed, weak-kneed I was
Unable to move, I let her pass
Awakened, I ran around
To meet her at the water fount
Lifting her eyebrows she smiled
And looked at me, so serene,
With her eyes of opal green
Taking courage I introduced myself
As Frans, said I had been on the shelf
Asked if we could meet another day
She said, "Yes, and my name is Gre"
After numerous dates, oh heavens above
We realized we were totally in love
With a Christian heritage to share
We became a happy pair.
In our mid-twenties feeling mature
We wanted marriage no other allure
Saw our Pastor and booked a hall
Married in February, had a ball!
Blessed with three daughters
No sons, I wasn't bothered
Grateful for their health and growth
Boyfriends came, we were not opposed
The entire world could see
We were a happy family.

Weathered disagreements and fights
As most healthy families
There were times, I confess
When I caused my wife stress
There were conflicts of needs
I had to learn how to please
God allowed me this wife
He helped us overcome all strife
Almost fifty years have gone by
Like aging wine, we're feeling high.
Dearest Grace my Love
Though older and silvery gray,
You are talented in every way.
In homemaking and baking
Especially in watercolor painting
I love you, dear, for your patience,
You have always been so gracious
Each time I see your opal green eyes,
I know with you I'm in paradise.

Happy Birthday, Sweetheart!

The Purpose Driven Life

It is all about our daily life
To be merry, no need to strive
For justice and a caring society
Or to show off our propriety?

Upon further reflection I found
That God said we are duty bound
God made us for a purpose
Gives direction, not to curse us

How will I know Gods plan for us
Reading the scriptures and thus
Find out that you are special too
And has things in store for you

I never thought of it that way
Knowing God created us from clay
Forming our bodies in full array
For which I am thankful every day

Lord being special is astounding
To be raised with love and care abounding
In society we be true and caring
Helping others with their needs and caring

We are grateful Lord that you are there
That you are in charge of us and care
For all our needs both great and small
In sickness or death, you're there for all

It is difficult to comprehend
To you, we are like a grain of sand
We cannot live up to all your laws
Still you love us despite our flaws

We desire to earn our keep
But are told the price is steep
God send his son to rescues us
From death; instead He died for us

Then if we cannot earn our keep
It is then that we must seek
To commit ourselves to our Lord and King
With our heart and soul to Him may cling

It's going to be a life long struggle
With ups and downs, some will grumble
Humbling ourselves to God and take
The road that Jesus took for our sake

Lord help us please to understand
For us to discover our talent
Having a special purpose for us in mind
Serving you without lament, and not be blind

Sharing with others about God and see
To live for Him and others in harmony
Supporting each other in needs and deeds
Forming communities that follow your creeds

May we discover your path for us
Following you Lord - our old nature crush
With joyful hearts we praise your name
Waiting for Jesus return to this earth again

To My Dear One

Want to get something off my chest
To be sure if I am you're very best
There is no reason to be afraid
You will never be betrayed

Its not that I am in the mood to confess
Just expressing my feelings and profess
Explain to you and record on this paper
My love for you, that will never waiver
I am write this down with my pen
Using ink, my way to say: amen

Years ago I wrote you a note
While traveling on a boat
Away from home, I felt amiss
Missed your presence and our bliss
Our oceans of love I wrote,
And on every wave a kiss
I'll go through rain, mud or slide
To be close and hold you by my side

While I am reading Shakespeare
It's becoming much more clear
My affection for you cannot compare
With some ordinary love affair
This wife of mine is sweeter than wine
She is a gift of God, therefore divine

Touchmark at Wedgewood

A Place where kinsfolk come together
Not in blood but like birds of a feather
We struck down to where it's warm
At Touchmark, because it has charm

Being full of accord and never bored
Just go and read the bulletin board
Dancing or exercise in the marquis
Or watching movies, witch much glee

We are a bit older but also bolder
Sometimes, we share our shoulder
If not to cry, then for pure joy
Respect for each and all we employ

We give comfort to each other
As a family of sisters and brothers
Wishing to beautify and honor those
That left us; In heaven may repose

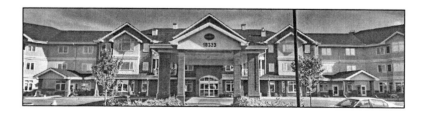

Touchmark Dining

A quote:
"We have a chef who is so adept in his art,
the aroma of his unsurpassing succulent
dishes will make you swoon with
pleasure and delight.
Our limpid tongue can never
Leave of savoring them."

Winston is our Chef
With his assistant Jeff
Everyday a celebration
Gourmet food with innovation

Winston's kitchen is his sanctum
His gourmet food to greet'em
Food presentation so enticing
Colourful and great in spicing

Diners expound with Ohs and Ahs
Tasting soup called vichyssoise
Every dish has eye appeal
Served with finesse so genteel

Every day, there are new delights
No doubt we will be satisfied
Nutritious food, no aphrodisiac
Might prevent a heart attack?

Portions are sized to prevent
The torment of possible flatulent
Touchmark dining Room,
With its beautiful décor
No black tie, do come in, *por favor.*

Touchmark Family

Touchmark a place of harmony
Residents and staff are family
A place of sharing and caring
Background stories comparing

Celebrating our joys and grief
Regardless of background or belief
Together we're like babes secluded
We are family no one is denuded

At Touchmark we are content
Our stay is not a punishment
We are happy here and not afraid
To make ready for heavens gate

Passed the world of status and affairs
Time for introspection and more prayers
We may laugh about our idiosyncrasies
With different background but at peace

Welcome to those over fifty-five
Join our fellowship while still alive
No more strive to make a living
Rest your laurels with thanksgiving

Traveling Alone

Riding a train through Italy
Met two women from Germany
Using their eyes to communicate
Lets go to Corfu, it was their bait

My mind ran amok, did intent
Follow suit, (must be God sent)
But little did I know
Prayers were offered long ago

By some-one and the Lord had heard
And sent his Angel, it seemed absurd
Lost my wallet, credit card and pass
Before the Lord, a lame Duck I was

A curtain dropped from my eyes
And I became much more wise
Passion may arise so naturally
Important to keep your sanctity

Vincent Van Gogh,
1853-1891

Vincent the dreamer
Had an artistic passion

His eyes translated scenes
Into ochre, rust, slate and red
His surroundings spoke to him
Of the colours all around

Loved literature - Latin
Dutch, French, English
His intellect helped him to see
The wonders of creation
His letters show an irresistible
Passion for describing creation
Images of intense beauty

A simple painting of a potato
Tells us about poverty
In the late 19th century
Feeling isolated from society
Vincent refused
To paint in a style expected
Causing grief and agitation
Occasionally became enraged

Felt rejected, took his life
No praise on Earth
But Angels shed their tears
For one whose brush glorified
God's colourful creation.

YMCA

The pool
An amputee
Swimming
Delighted

Exercising
Without pain
Swimming
At six am

No competion
Pretending, its my pool
Dreaming away
What is to come
Memory of my past

Back packing
Running
Some times wining
Opportunity, too
To be thankful
For a new day

More dreams
Water hypnotic
Swimming
On the waves
Will prevent
An early grave
By God,s grace

Epilogue

Facing the Darkness

In September 2005, my wife, Grace, and I, moved to Touchmark at Wedgewood – a resort style accommodation - which we are now happy to call home. When we moved there I was both excited and apprehensive. Change is a little tough sometimes, not to mention both Grace and I got a bit of a shock when we realized that at 76 and 78 years of age, we were the 'kids' on the block. We had expected to meet some younger people but most were over 80 and a few had conquered the 90+ hurdle.

It was a tough decision to leave our former home, but with both of us having health issues we decided that a 1500 square foot condominium was too much for us to look after. Grace, brought up to be a hard worker, could never settle until everything was in its place and all was spic and span. It bothered me a lot to see her toiling so hard, looking after the place and caring for me. She was ready to move. We both were. There were times when I wondered what we were doing. But soon we settled and now I believe God knew his restless child (me) would need help in his later days.

I was born May 24, 1929 and physically, I am in good health and have adapted well over the years despite my below the knee amputation. However, I have recently learned that I am in the early stages, of Alzheimer's.

Nearly 5 years ago, I took a course on creative writing. I soon discovered I had difficulty following the readings of my fellow storywriters. So now and then I would ask one of them if I could get a copy of his or her story. I needed to read it on my own steam in order to fathom the content. Since English is my second language, I started to wonder if that was the issue or could it be age?

Perhaps I was in denial. I started to justify and contemplate the reasons for me not 'getting it' when people spoke to me or read aloud in my presence. The Dutch language has changed over time. So after living in Canada for so long, I started to feel more comfortable speaking and writing English, although there were still times when I needed clarification. Was the language crossover the problem? Or was something else happening to me?

Since our move to Touchmark, I have watched and have been in contact with other residents who I soon learned had advanced Alzheimer's disease. As I started making friends I found myself meeting with these people and I wondered about my own situation. Was I at that stage of my life, even though I was one of the younger residents?

A few years ago, after dealing with some retention issues, I decided to make contact with a Neuropsychological specialist. After an initial assessment, he checked my memory through a series of cognitive impairment tests. The results indicated my worst fears - the early onset of dementia.

During the first few days following my diagnosis I had a difficult time adjusting. It made me wonder. How do I face the future? Do I quit writing? Do I have to stop driving my car? How do I go about meeting my friends and other persons, when I cannot find the appropriate words to express myself? All these thoughts came to me and I was inclined to stay away from others fearing I would look and sound a fool. What about my wife who depends on me? Maybe she wouldn't be able to look after me, when the disease progresses to the later stages. I couldn't bear to think about that.

I prayed and asked God for direction. Then I started reading his Word. In Proverbs 3: 5-6 I found my answer: Trust in the LORD with all your heart and lean not on your own understanding; in all your ways submit to him, and he will make your paths straight.

It was then I decided to carry on and enjoy my life with Grace. My children would be my pride and joy and getting together with our friends would rank high on our to-do list.

At present I do quite well communicating and remembering, although I do have my moments and I try to find ways to compensate. Most people with whom I have contact have not noticed my condition. I usually let whoever I am speaking with do most of the talking, while I nod a lot, use simple words, and try to keep the discussion short.

But there are times – frustrating and maddening moments, when I cannot find the words that I know would describe my thoughts. My writing has become much slower. Words used to flow like the springtime sap but now I hesitate and fumble a little too much for my liking. When I am looking for the right words,

I ask my wife, bless her patient heart, or I grab a dictionary. But sometimes a dictionary does not help because I need to know how a word begins. If the word will not come alive in my mind, then I am stuck. If dear Gracie cannot help me, I visit the friendly secretary at the front desk and ask her for the spelling or for a better word. She is always ready to help jog my memory.

Family and close friends are aware of my difficulty and challenges; they will wait patiently for me to find the right words when a particular thought won't process. Sometimes I just sit and think and wonder how long it will take my brain to catch up and sort out my thoughts.

Driving is a concern. So far I have been able to drive anywhere, and often use a map to be sure how to get to my destination in my own town. Twice I got lost and much to my chagrin, I had to stop and ask for directions! I recall once when this happened to me, a part of a song came to mind. "I once was lost, but now am found!" Good thing I haven't lost my sense of humour yet!

Gracie is my confidant and clarifier [thank goodness]. Sometimes even going for breakfast in our community dining room is a challenge these days because I forget. I might hear 'scrambled eggs' yet cannot remember what that is.

But Gracie sticks pretty close to me and interprets what's on the menu. Other times I might get side-tracked from a task when Mother Nature calls. Three minutes in the bathroom, and I have already forgotten what I was doing or planning on doing. So far my solution is to walk around the room, and retrace my steps. Sometimes I get back on track. Gracie is often surprised that I forget such simple things, but then the two of us consider it funny. I wonder if, in the future, I will still laugh at my own foibles.

Staying at home probably is not the wisest choice for those struggling with dementia but it seems to be a protective mechanism of sorts for me. I feel at peace if I do not have to have a conversation with anyone. I do not have to worry about finding certain sensible words or how to answer a question.

As it is, I spend endless hours on my computer hunting for words that escape me or I grab the dictionary in a desperate search for what I want to say. My short term memory seems to be getting worse and I find I can forget things in a mere moment. Some days it is just easier for me to retreat inwardly and communicate with self. No one knows then, what I am juggling with in my brain.

In 2009 I wrote and published a book called Journal of a Dutch Immigrant. For the past two years I have had the privilege of setting up a table now and again at Indigo and Chapters bookstores and the occasional local farmer's market. I found this a great way to sell books and meet my readers face to face. I used to love entering into conversations and utilizing my past experience in sales. But things have changed. Now if I do dare venture out to sell some books, my approach is a little different. When interested customers ask me questions, I try to side track them by suggesting they read the blurb at the back of the book. So far I have managed not to come off sounding like I don't know what I am talking about. By telling the listener a sad story about my past that happens to be explained in my book, I can cope with the face to face interactions and usually answer their questions.

One Sunday morning during a church service, I recall singing that fairly familiar chorus - My Life is in You Lord. For some reason it was so helpful for what I was facing; both the words and the tune really struck a chord. I forgot my concern about the future. It reminded me to remember Who and what my life was all about. No matter the eventuality, the Lord was with me and I with Him. Funny how that day sticks in my mind. After that reassuring song, we headed home. I recall reading a book while Gracie made our dinner. I love the smell of her cooking – always have. It was such a peaceful time, complete with good food, a good nap and the best company; God soothed my soul and my fears that day.

Over the past 50 years I have travelled to different countries often ending up in places where I should not be. But God was on the job. And I thank Him for going with me and protecting me. He must have brooded over this wanderlust child who would one day need help. God, in His infinite wisdom, sent angels to keep me from the evil one, who often tried to lead me to places where angels feared to tread!

Life's treasures, I have discovered, consist of family, friends and experiences. In my younger days, I spent a lot of time exploring and experiencing God's amazing creation. I did a lot of cycling short and long distances; running either marathons or just for the fun of it; backpacking in the mountains; swimming and more. Even when I lost my left leg below the knee following a horrific vehicle accident in 1987, I managed to remain active. Although I was no longer able to cycle and run, I was still able to swim. It took two years to fully recover but I was determined to keep fit. I returned to the YMCA swimming pool three times a week, starting at 6.30 in the morning. I still swim 40 minutes each day and cover 100 meters. When I swim I see it as a place where I can think and enjoy my wellness. I thank God for giving me the strength to do so and the perseverance to rise and conquer the tragedy of my accident.

I might not understand what is happening to me now and why the road ahead looks so grim and dark. I also know the path ahead will be a challenge for both Gracie, my children and for me. I expect to encounter some difficult times in the near future. But I am trusting God to look after us. It might take a few years, until I leave this earth; maybe more. But I am not afraid. I am secure in knowing that I am heading to heaven and God has promised me that there, I will enjoy an everlasting and beautiful, peaceful place. He is holding my hand, helping me to face the darkness, and reassuring me that it is well with my soul. My mind may wander sometimes, but my heart is fixed on God...

Alzheimer

Something new
Been informed
Memory is short
Still know the past
Forget the future
I live for the day

Psalm Twenty Three

The Lord is my shepherd
I shall not want
He makes me lie down
In green pastures
Even though I walk
Through a dark valley

I am not afraid
God will take care of me
And will comfort me
He has promised me
That there will be a day
I will dwell in the
House of the Lord

A wonderful future
No need to cry
But will re-choice
In my God.

CPSIA information can be obtained at www.ICGtesting.com
Printed in the USA
LVOW081922051012

301700LV00005B/8/P

9 781770 694354